STATISTICS IN CLINICAL PRACTICE

STATISTICS IN CLINICAL PRACTICE

DAVID COGGON
MA PhD DM FRCP FFOM

Reader in Occupational and Environmental Medicine
MRC Environmental Epidemiology Unit
University of Southampton

BMJ
Publishing
Group

First published in 1995
by the BMJ Publishing Group, BMA House, Tavistock Square, London WC1H 9JR

British Library Cataloguing in Publication Data

A catalogue record for this book is available from the British Library

ISBN 0-7279-0907-X

Printed and bound in Great Britain by
Latimer Trend & Company Ltd., Plymouth

Contents

Foreword

The bad news for many medical students and doctors is that these days one cannot practise medicine well without some understanding of statistics. Most papers in medical journals use statistical techniques to summarise or interpret observations, and even at clinical meetings it is difficult to escape at least occasional reference to standard deviations and P values. A doctor with no knowledge of statistics is unable to evaluate much of the scientific information that is crucial to the optimal care of patients. This dependence on statistical methods is reflected in undergraduate and postgraduate curricula.

The good news is that doctors need not be mathematicians to use statistics. In the same way that a report of a plasma creatinine concentration can be interpreted and acted on without a detailed understanding of the laboratory methods underlying the assay, so it is not necessary for a doctor to understand all the mathematical intricacies of a statistical calculation in order to apply its results. Just as we normally trust the biochemist to use an appropriate analytical method, so we may put faith in medical statisticians to get their sums right. It helps if doctors can carry out simpler tasks such as calculating means and standard deviations, but more important is the ability to communicate with statisticians—to formulate a problem in such a way that a statistician can advise on an appropriate analytical method; to recognise and assess any biological assumptions that are inherent in the statistical analysis; and particularly to understand the results of statistical calculations when they are presented.

This book is aimed at doctors and medical students who view statistics as a necessary evil. It is not intended as a manual for those wishing to carry out their own statistical analyses beyond the simple summarising of data that might be required for a clinical meeting. Rather, it sets out to explain the principles of statistics that must be understood in order to read journals and practise clinical medicine competently, and it does this without using any mathematics beyond the level needed for school leavers. For readers who prefer a more detailed and mathematical approach, many other texts are available, some of which are listed on page 112. The book divides into three sections. Chapters 1 to 3 are concerned with descriptive statistics used to summarise data numerically and graphically so that they can be better understood and communicated. Chapter 4 introduces the concept of probability and gives examples of its applications in clinical practice. Chapters 5 to 9 deal with statistical inference and the methods by which general conclusions can be drawn from observations made on samples of patients or clinical material. Principles are illustrated with examples from many different fields of medicine and, to help reinforce readers' understanding, questions are included at the end of each chapter with answers starting on page 104. The examples and questions are constructed to demonstrate particular teaching points, and to achieve this some use fictitious data. However, all are intended to be realistic.

DAVID COGGON
June 1995

1 Types of data

Table 1.1 shows an extract from data on a consecutive series of births at a district general hospital over a 12 month period. It contains information that might be useful as part of an audit of the maternity service for the district. For example, it tells us something about the level of activity of the service, how work is apportioned between various consultants and the general practitioner unit, and the nature of the hospital's patient mix. As presented, however, the data are difficult to digest. Just glancing at the table we get an impression that roughly half the babies are boys and that most mothers stay in hospital for two to four days after delivery, but much of the information is relatively inaccessible. From the full data set it might not be immediately obvious whether one consultant cared for more mothers from lower social classes or kept patients in hospital for a longer time than the average. An obstetrician who went to an audit meeting and presented 20 slides in the format of table 1.1 would not be thanked by colleagues.

Much more helpful would be to summarise the data, presenting only the information that was relevant to the audit exercise—for example, the numbers of mothers looked after by each consultant and their social class distribution. This process of summarising data is achieved by use of *descriptive statistics*. The summary may be numerical—the mean birth weight of the babies, for example—or graphical—as in a plot showing the relation of birth weight to the parity of the mother. Graphical summaries allow a lot of information to be assimilated rapidly, but numerical summaries are often more precise and have the advantage that they can be communicated in spoken as well as written form. The choice between numerical and graphical summary depends on the type of data under consideration, the information that is to be abstracted, and the circumstances in which it is to be communicated (in a written report, at a meeting, over the telephone, and so on). To some extent it is a matter of personal taste.

1

Table 1.1 Extract from data on a consecutive series of births at a district general hospital over a 12 month period

Consultant	Mother's age	Mother's social class	No. of previous pregnancies	Sex of baby	Birth weight (g)	Singleton or multiple birth	Mother's length of stay after delivery (days)
GP unit	31	II	1	F	3460	S	2
Miss White	25	IIIM	1	M	3740	S	3
Miss White	24	IIIN	0	F	2790	S	4
Mr Green	30	II	1	F	3340	S	2
Mr Black	28	IIIN	1	M	3920	S	1
Miss White	24	II	0	F	3250	S	3
GP unit	26	IV	1	F	2875	S	2
Mr Black	23	IIIN	0	M	2945	S	4
Mr Green	26	II	1	F	3100	S	2
Mr Green	33	II	1	M	2910	S	1
Miss White	25	V	1	F	3455	S	2
GP unit	20	IIIN	0	M	3795	S	4
GP unit	30	II	1	F	4070	S	2
Mr Black	32	IIIN	1	M	2580	M	10
Mr Black	32	IIIN	1	M	2655	M	10
Miss White	24	IIIN	0	F	2510	S	4

The techniques used to summarise data, whether numerically or in graphical form, are determined by the nature of the data. It is helpful, therefore, to review the types of data that are commonly encountered in medical practice. As we shall see later, this classification of data is relevant not only to their summary by descriptive statistics, but also in the approaches adopted to statistical inference (see chapter 5).

Nominal, ordinal, and quantitative data

Table 1.1 contains information about eight items of information for each birth. These *variables* fall into several distinct types. The sex of the baby and the identity of the supervising consultant are examples of *nominal* data. Each birth belongs to one of a set of mutually exclusive categories (male/female, Miss White/Mr Green/ Mr Black/GP unit). Moreover, these categories have no inherent order. For example, there is no special reason to place Mr Green between Miss White and Mr Black—we could quite reasonably list them in some other sequence.

The social class of the mother also belongs to a set of mutually exclusive categories, but in this case the categories do have a natural order:

I	Professional occupations
II	Intermediate occupations
IIIN	Skilled non-manual occupations
IIIM	Skilled manual occupations
IV	Semi-skilled occupations
V	Unskilled occupations

In listing the classes it would not make sense to place professional women between unskilled and semi-skilled workers. Data such as social class that fall into an ordered series of three or more categories are termed *ordinal*.* Another example of ordinal data is the grading

---

* A categorical variable that can take only two possible values is described as *binary* and is always classed as nominal.

of muscle strength sometimes used by neurologists:

0 No active contraction
1 Visible or palpable contraction without active movement
2 Movement with gravity eliminated
3 Movement against gravity
4 Movement against gravity plus resistance
5 Normal power

Although it is conventional to label social classes and levels of muscle strength numerically, these numbers tell us only about their rank order. A muscle strength of grade 4 cannot necessarily be interpreted as twice grade 2. It is simply more than grade 3, which in turn is more than grade 2.

In contrast, data such as birth weight and mother's age are truly *quantitative*. Such quantitative data can be further classified according to whether they are *discrete* or *continuous*. Discrete quantitative data can take only a limited number of possible values. For example, the number of previous pregnancies must be a whole number, and these days will rarely exceed 12. On the other hand, birth weight can lie anywhere in a continuum from less than 1500 g to more than 4500 g. Of course, this continuity depends in practice on the precision with which the weights are recorded. If measurements were made only to the nearest kilogram, the variable would effectively be discrete. The borderline between discrete and continuous data is somewhat arbitrary, but variables can reasonably be considered continuous if the number of possible values is more than 20.

Univariate, bivariate, and multivariate data

One way of looking at the data in table 1.1 is to consider the variables one at a time. For example, we might start by concentrating solely on the birth weights and examine their distribution for all of the babies. This analysis would be based on

4

Box 1.A   Birth weights (in grams) from a consecutive series of babies born in a district general hospital

3460	3100
3740	2910
2790	3455
3340	3795
3920	4070
3250	2580
2875	2655
2945	2510

Box 1.B   Sexes of a consecutive series of babies born in a district general hospital

F	F
M	M
F	F
F	M
M	F
F	M
F	M
M	F

the subset of data of the form shown in box 1.A and would be classed as *univariate* as it incorporates a single item of information for each birth. Similarly, the subset of data in box 1.B concerning the sex of the babies is univariate.

5

Table 1.2 Sex and birth weight (in grams) of a consecutive
series of babies born in a district general hospital

Sex	Birth weight	Sex	Birth weight
F	3460	F	3100
M	3740	M	2910
F	2790	F	3455
F	3340	M	3795
M	3920	F	4070
F	3250	M	2580
F	2875	M	2655
M	2945	F	2510

Looking independently at the sex and birth weight of the babies tells us nothing about how the two are related to each other—for example, whether the boys tended to be heavier than the girls. To answer this question we need data in the form shown in table 1.2. These are *bivariate* data comprising two linked pieces of information—the sex and the birth weight—for each baby.

More complex analyses might look at the interrelation of three, four, or even more variables using *multivariate* data. Table 1.1 is an example of a multivariate data set containing eight linked items of information for each birth.

Chapter 2 describes techniques for summarising univariate data, and chapter 3 deals with the summary of bivariate and multivariate data.

Questions

1.1 Classify the following variables according to whether they are nominal, ordinal, discrete quantitative, or continuous quantitative.

(a) Systolic blood pressure, measured to the nearest mm Hg, in a series of patients admitted to hospital with myocardial infarction.

(b) Blood cholesterol level, measured to the nearest 0·1 mmol/l, in a series of men attending a health promotion clinic.

(c) Number of previous blood transfusions in a series of renal transplant patients.

(d) Blood group.

(e) Antibody titres to cytomegalovirus (measured to one of eight possible levels).

(f) Ethnic origin (classified as Afro-Caribbean, white, Chinese, Indian, or other).

(g) Educational level (classified as primary, secondary, or higher).

(h) Number of sexual partners in the past month in a series of patients attending a clinic for sexually transmitted diseases.

(i) Smoking habit (classified as ever smoked or never smoked).

(j) Cause of death (classified as cancer, cardiovascular disease, respiratory disease, or other).

(k) Grade of surgeon (classified as senior house officer, registrar, senior registrar, or consultant).

1.2 In a survey carried out at a general practitioner's surgery, information was collected on each patient's sex, age, presenting complaint, and whether any medication was prescribed. How many bivariate combinations can be made up from these variables?

2 Summarising univariate data

Nominal data

Box 2.A lists the diagnoses of a series of patients admitted to a surgical unit. The diagnostic categories have no natural order, so these are nominal data.

The simplest way to summarise such data numerically is by a *frequency count*, giving the number of patients with each diagnosis (table 2.1). Alternatively, or in addition, one can calculate the *proportion* or percentage of patients in each diagnostic category. The advantage of proportions is that they facilitate comparisons with other series in which the total number of patients is different (table 2.2). However, if proportions are quoted without frequency counts, it is helpful at least to indicate the total number of observations on which they are based. A statement that "10% of

Table 2.1 Frequency count summarising the data presented in box 2.A, and showing proportions of patients for each diagnostic category

Diagnosis	No of patients	Proportion of patients (%)
Cholelithiasis	12	25
Inguinal hernia	9	19
Cancer of colon	9	19
Duodenal ulcer	4	8
Cancer of pancreas	4	8
Cancer of rectum	3	6
Gastric ulcer	2	4
Cancer of stomach	2	4
Cancer of oesophagus	2	4
Oesophageal stricture	1	2
All diagnoses	48	100

Box 2.A Diagnoses of a series of 48 patients admitted to a surgical unit

Gastric ulcer	Inguinal hernia
Cholelithiasis	Cholelithiasis
Cholelithiasis	Cancer of colon
Cancer of rectum	Oesophageal stricture
Cancer of stomach	Cholelithiasis
Duodenal ulcer	Cancer of colon
Cancer of colon	Cancer of pancreas
Inguinal hernia	Duodenal ulcer
Duodenal ulcer	Cholelithiasis
Inguinal hernia	Gastric ulcer
Inguinal hernia	Inguinal hernia
Cholelithiasis	Cancer of pancreas
Cancer of colon	Cancer of colon
Cholelithiasis	Cancer of rectum
Cancer of colon	Cholelithiasis
Cancer of pancreas	Cancer of stomach
Cholelithiasis	Cancer of oesophagus
Cancer of oesophagus	Cholelithiasis
Inguinal hernia	Cancer of pancreas
Duodenal ulcer	Inguinal hernia
Cholelithiasis	Cancer of colon
Cholelithiasis	Inguinal hernia
Cancer of colon	Cancer of rectum
Inguinal hernia	Cancer of colon

patients undergoing hip replacement were treated privately" carries more weight in a comparison if it is 10% of 200 patients rather than 10% of 20 patients.

Proportions should not be given unwarranted precision. If altogether there are only 30 observations then it is clearly inappropriate to quote percentages to four decimal places. As a rule of thumb, if there are fewer than 100 observations in total then it is not worth calculating percentages to more than the nearest whole number. Because of rounding errors, individual percentages may sum to slightly more or less than 100 (as in table 2.2).

9

Table 2.2   Comparison of diagnoses in two series of surgical patients

Diagnosis	Proportion of patients (%)	
	First series (n = 48)	Second series (n = 71)
Cholelithiasis	25	13
Inguinal hernia	19	14
Cancer of colon	19	17
Duodenal ulcer	8	8
Cancer of pancreas	8	14
Cancer of rectum	6	11
Gastric ulcer	4	4
Cancer of stomach	4	11
Cancer of oesophagus	4	4
Oesophageal stricture	2	0
Appendix abscess	0	3

Note that although percentages are used for the comparison, the total numbers of patients in each series (n = 48 and n = 71) are also given. Because of rounding errors each column of percentages totals to 99 rather than 100

Table 2.3   Frequency of deaths from different types of accidental injury in male farmers aged 20–64 in England and Wales during 1979–80 and 1982–90

Type of accident	Number of deaths
Transport accidents	
Off-road motor vehicle accidents	32
Animal transport accidents	12
Poisoning	
Pesticides	3
Gases	7
Injury by animals	17
Injury by falling object	30
Injury by machinery	127
Injury by firearms	20
Injury by electric current	28

Subdivisions of different categories of accidents are grouped together

When frequency counts and proportions are presented in tabular form, the order of the different nominal categories is optional. One approach might be to list them in order of descending frequency, as in table 2.1, but this is not essential. When some of the categories have subdivisions it makes sense to group the subdivisions together, as in table 2.3.

10

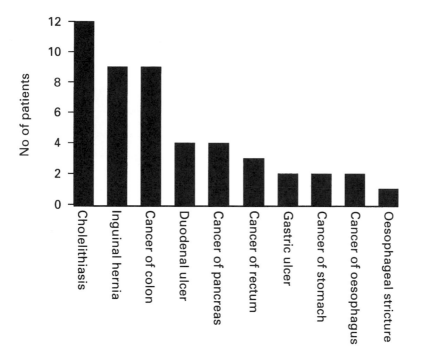

Figure 2.1 *Bar chart based on data summarised in table 2.1*
Each diagnosis is represented by a separate bar, the height of which corresponds to the frequency of the diagnosis

Bar charts and pie charts

Nominal data can be summarised graphically by bar charts or pie charts. In a bar chart (fig 2.1) there is one bar for each nominal category, with the height of the bar corresponding to the frequency count of the category. The values of frequency counts or proportions, or both, should be indicated—for example, by a scale, as in figure 2.1. All of the bars should be of equal width and they are normally separated from each other.

Sometimes, where the differences between frequency counts are small in comparison with the absolute values of frequencies, the

11

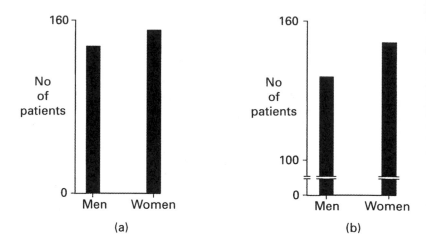

Figure 2.2 *Effect of breaking the scale in a bar chart*

Figures (a) and (b) show the distribution, according to sex, of patients attending a general practice because of low back pain. The effect of breaking the axis, as in (b), is to exaggerate differences between categories. Note that breaks are shown both in the scale and in the bars

scale of a bar chart is broken, as in figure 2.2. The effect is to exaggerate the differences between categories. This technique is best avoided, but if it is used, the breaks in the scale and bars must be clearly indicated.

A pie chart (fig 2.3) is an effective way of demonstrating the proportions of observations falling in different nominal categories. Each category is represented by a segment of a circle (a slice of the pie), the area of the segment corresponding to the proportion of observations in the category. The order in which segments are arranged around the circle is arbitrary.

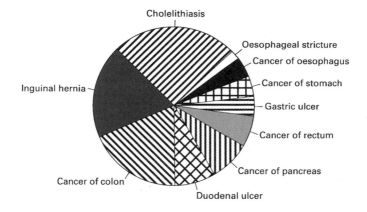

Figure 2.3 *Pie chart based on the data summarised in table 2.1*
Each diagnosis is represented by a segment of the circle, the area of which corresponds to its frequency as a proportion of all diagnoses

Ordinal data

The methods of summarising ordinal data are similar to those used for nominal data, except that tables and charts should display the categories of an ordinal variable in their natural sequence. For example, figure 2.4 shows different ways of summarising data on the severity of pneumoconiosis in a population of coal miners.

Quantitative data

A set of quantitative measurements can be summarised numerically by measures of central tendency (where the "middle" of the distribution of measurements lies) and of dispersion (how spread out the measurements are).

13

(a) *Table showing a frequency count*

Grade of pneumoconiosis	Number of miners	Proportion of miners (%)
Category 0	38	17·3
Category 1	56	25·5
Category 2	73	33·2
Category 3	53	24·1

(b) *Bar chart*

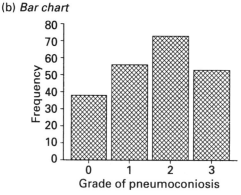

(c) *Pie chart*

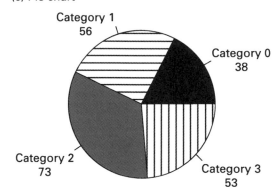

Figure 2.4 *Methods of summarising the distribution of pneumoconiosis grades in a series of coal miners*

In each case the grades of pneumoconiosis are set out in their natural order. Grades of pneumoconiosis are classified by comparison of chest radiographs with standard films

---

Box 2.B   Calculation of the mean and median of 15 blood glucose levels

In a series of 15 patients fasting blood glucose levels (mmol/l) were recorded as follows:

5·8, 4·3, 25·9, 5·2, 6·1, 3·9, 4·4, 5·6, 5·3, 4·5, 4·6, 3·8, 5·1, 5·4, 4·6

The mean is obtained by adding together all of the measurements and then dividing by the number of measurements. Thus it is given by:

(5·8 + 4·3 + 25·9 + 5·2 + 6·1 + 3·9 + 4·4 + 5·6 + 5·3 + 4·5 + 4·6 + 3·8 + 5·1 + 5·4 + 4·6)/15 = 94·5/15 = 6·3

To calculate the median, the 15 measurements are first ranked in ascending order:

3·8, 3·9, 4·3, 4·4, 4·5, 4·6, 4·6, <u>5·1</u>, 5·2, 5·3, 5·4, 5·6, 5·8, 6·1, 25·9

The median is then given by the middle value in the ranking: 5·1.

Statistical packages for computers include routines for deriving means and medians.

Central tendency

The most familiar measure of central tendency is the *mean* or average of the observations. This is calculated by adding together all of the measurements and then dividing the total by the number of measurements. Thus the mean of the 15 blood glucose levels in box 2.B is 6.3 mmol/l. The mean of a discrete quantitative variable need not necessarily take one of the discrete values of the variable. The oft-quoted average of 2·4 children in a family is acceptable even though it is not a whole number.

The other measure of central tendency in common usage is the *median*. This is derived by ranking all of the measurements in ascending order and then selecting the middle value (box 2.B).

15

Box 2.C   Calculation of the median of an even number of measurements

In a series of 20 patients from a renal unit, haemoglobin levels (mg/100 ml) were recorded as follows:

8·4, 11·9, 6·3, 8·2, 9·5, 9·0, 7·6, 9·0, 10·1, 9·8, 8·9, 10·4, 7·6, 8·8, 11·5, 10·6, 8·2, 8·7, 9·0, 8·8

To calculate the median, we first rank the measurements in ascending order:

6·3, 7·6, 7·6, 8·2, 8·2, 8·4, 8·7, 8·8, 8·8, 8·9, 9·0, 9·0, 9·0, 9·5, 9·8, 10·1, 10·4, 10·6, 11·5, 11·9

We then calculate the mean of the middle two values in the ranking:

$(8·9 + 9·0)/2 = 8·95$

Where there are an even number of measurements in a data set, the median is the mean of the middle two measurements in the ranking (box 2.C).

Note that the mean can be strongly influenced by outlying values of a variable. For example, the mean of the glucose levels in box 2.B is 6·3 mmol/l. Without the outlying value of 25·9 it would come down to 4·9 mmol/l. The median of 5·1 mmol/l, on the other hand, is changed much less by exclusion of the outlier, reducing only by 0·25 mmol/l.*

Dispersion

The simplest measure of dispersion is the *range* of a variable—that is, the difference between its highest and lowest values. In practice, it is usually quoted by stating these extreme values explicitly—range 3·8 to 25·9 mmol/l, for example. By definition, the range, like the mean, is sensitive to any outlying observations, which is a particular disadvantage when outliers may be "rogue results" arising from

---

* These calculations with exclusion of an outlier are presented to illustrate a point. When analysing data it is sometimes tempting to exclude outlying values that do not fit the overall pattern. However, such a step is usually incorrect and should not be taken without good justification.

16

Box 2.D Calculation of the interquartile range for the blood glucose measurements listed in box 2.B

Firstly, the 15 measurements are ranked in ascending order:

3·8, 3·9, 4·3, <u>4·4</u>, 4·5, 4·6, 4·6, 5·1, 5·2, 5·3, 5·4, <u>5·6</u>, 5·8, 6·1, 25·9

The lower quartile is the value one quarter of the way up the ranked list: 4·4 mmol/l.

The upper quartile is the value three quarters of the way up the ranked list: 5·6 mmol/l.

The interquartile range is the difference between the upper and lower quartiles: $5·6 - 4·4 = 1·2$ mmol/l.

In this example with 15 measurements, definition of the quartiles is straightforward, but with other numbers of observations it is sometimes necessary to take a weighted average of the two measurements lying either side of the quarter way mark in the ranking and of the two measurements either side of the three quarter way mark (rather as the median of an even number of measurements is the average of the two central values). Fortunately, this is normally done automatically by a computer program.

---

measurement errors. The problem can be overcome by instead using the *interquartile range*. This is calculated by ranking all of the measurements in ascending order and identifying the lower and upper *quartiles*—the values lying a quarter and three quarters of the way up the ranked list (box 2.D). The interquartile range is the difference between the upper and lower quartiles, and like the range is usually quoted by giving its extremes—interquartile range 4·4 to 5·6 mmol/l, for example.

The measure of dispersion most often encountered in medical practice is the *standard deviation*, definition of which is rather more complicated. Firstly, the mean of the variable is derived. Next, the difference between each measurement and this mean (its deviation from the mean) is calculated. Each deviation is then squared. The squared deviations are summed for the whole data set and divided by the number of measurements minus one to obtain a quantity known as their *variance*. The standard deviation is the square root

17

Table 2.4 Calculation of the standard deviation for the blood glucose measurements listed in box 2.B

Measurement	Deviation	Squared deviation
5·8	$5·8 - 6·3 = -0·5$	$(-0·5)^2 = 0·25$
4·3	$4·3 - 6·3 = -2·0$	$(-2·0)^2 = 4·00$
25·9	$25·9 - 6·3 = +19·6$	$(+19·6)^2 = 384·16$
5·2	$5·2 - 6·3 = -1·1$	$(-1·1)^2 = 1·21$
6·1	$6·1 - 6·3 = -0·2$	$(-0·2)^2 = 0·04$
3·9	$3·9 - 6·3 = -2·4$	$(-2·4)^2 = 5·76$
4·4	$4·4 - 6·3 = -1·9$	$(-1·9)^2 = 3·61$
5·6	$5·6 - 6·3 = -0·7$	$(-0·7)^2 = 0·49$
5·3	$5·3 - 6·3 = -1·0$	$(-1·0)^2 = 1·00$
4·5	$4·5 - 6·3 = -1·8$	$(-1·8)^2 = 3·24$
4·6	$4·6 - 6·3 = -1·7$	$(-1·7)^2 = 2·89$
3·8	$3·8 - 6·3 = -2·5$	$(-2·5)^2 = 6·25$
5·1	$5·1 - 6·3 = -1·2$	$(-1·2)^2 = 1·44$
5·4	$5·4 - 6·3 = -0·9$	$(-0·9)^2 = 0·81$
4·6	$4·6 - 6·3 = -1·7$	$(-1·7)^2 = 2·89$

The mean of the 15 measurements in box 2.B is 6·3. The variance or mean squared deviation is given by: $(0·25 + 4·00 + 384·16 + 1·21 + 0·04 + 5·76 + 3·61 + 0·49 + 1·00 + 3·24 + 2·89 + 6·25 + 1·44 + 0·81 + 2·89)/(15 - 1) = 418·04/14 = 29·86$. The standard deviation is the square root of the variance: $\sqrt{(29·86)} = 5·5$ mmol/l

of the variance. The definition can perhaps be better understood from the example in table 2.4.†

In practice, standard deviations are normally obtained by the push of a button on a calculator or computer (as are the other statistics described in this chapter). However, an appreciation of their definition is necessary if the results of the computation are to be meaningful. It is not too difficult to see that the more dispersed a set of measurements, the bigger their deviations from the mean will be, and therefore the larger their standard deviation. The reason for adopting this particular measure of dispersion (rather than simply calculating the average deviation, for example) is that it has convenient mathematical properties, especially in the

† Many calculators and spreadsheets allow derivation of two standard deviations. One, denoted by S_x or σ_{n-1}, is calculated according to the definition given here; this is the one that is normally used. The other, denoted by σ_x or σ_n, entails dividing the sum of the squared deviations by the number of measurements rather than this number minus one. When the number of measurements is large there is almost no difference between σ_{n-1} and σ_n. The reason for preferring σ_{n-1} lies in the mathematics of statistical inference: defined in this way, the standard deviation of a sample of measurements gives a better estimate of the standard deviation of the population from which the sample was taken.

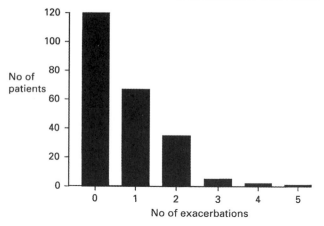

Figure 2.5 *Bar chart showing frequency of exacerbations requiring treatment with oral steroids in a group of asthmatic patients followed over 12 months*

context of statistical inference. The nature of these advantages need not concern us here, but it is important to be aware that standard deviation and variance measure the spread of a distribution. It should be noted that a standard deviation has the same units as the measurements from which it is derived. For example, in table 2.4 it is measured in mmol/l.

Graphical representation

The numerical summaries that have been described above can be applied equally to discrete and continuous quantitative data. The techniques for summarising quantitative data graphically, however, differ according to whether they are discrete or continuous. As for nominal and ordinal data, the distribution of discrete quantitative data can be displayed in the form of a bar chart. For example, figure 2.5 shows the number of exacerbations requiring treatment with oral steroids in a group of asthmatic patients followed for 12 months. The frequency of each number of exacerbations is represented by a separate bar centred on that number.

19

These data are systolic blood pressures (mm Hg) measured in 60 men attending a health promotion clinic:

140	109	144	162	115	125
131	164	155	178	162	144
133	133	121	135	142	130
113	137	128	142	167	134
166	146	113	150	128	117
160	154	139	135	117	124
143	118	105	107	158	144
129	120	148	139	172	127
133	129	174	153	141	131
156	152	130	148	151	125

Trying to summarise the data in a bar chart would produce a cumbersome plot, the left-handed end of which is shown;

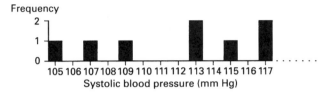

A much more useful graphical representation is obtained with a histogram:

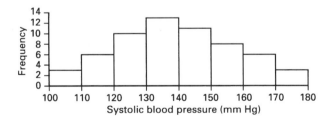

Pressures that are an exact multiple of 10 are here counted in the higher of the two rectangles to which they might be assigned. Thus, a value of 140 is counted as 140–150 and a value of 150 as 150–160.

Figure 2.6 *Histograms*

With continuous data, bar charts are inappropriate. Figure 2.6 shows the systolic blood pressures of 60 patients attending a

20

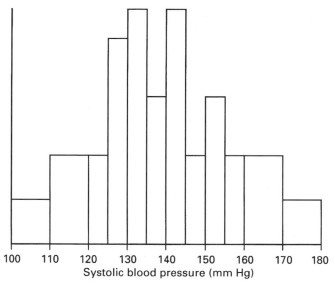

Systolic blood pressure (mm Hg)

Figure 2.7 *Histogram with unequal intervals*

This is an alternative plot of the data in figure 2.6. Intervals of 10 mm Hg have been used at the extremes and 5 mm Hg intervals have been used elsewhere. It is the area of rectangles – not their height – that corresponds to the frequency count

health promotion clinic. The values range from 105 mm Hg to 178 mm Hg. If we tried to depict these data in a bar chart we would obtain a cumbersome plot, the left-hand end of which is shown in figure 2.6. Almost all of the bars would be one unit high, and between the bars there would be wide gaps. We might just as well have stuck with the raw data in the original table.

The answer to this problem is to partition the range of blood pressures into intervals and plot the frequency with which pressures were recorded in each interval as a *histogram*. In a histogram each interval is represented by a rectangle, the width of which corresponds to the range of the interval and the area of which represents the frequency of measurements within the interval. The intervals need not all be equal (fig 2.7), but note that where they are not, it is the area of the rectangle and not its height which corresponds to the frequency count. Unlike in a bar chart, the rectangles are contiguous.

21

If the data from figure 2.6 are replotted with intervals that are too narrow (2 mm Hg) we end up with an unhelpful picture similar to a bar chart:

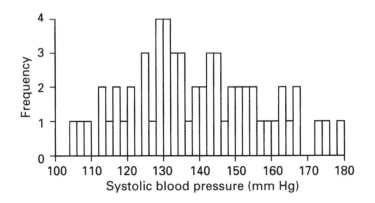

If the intervals are too large (25 mm Hg), useful detail is lost:

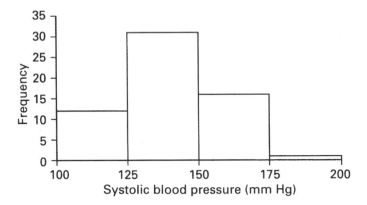

Figure 2.8 *Effect of varying the numbers of intervals in a histogram*

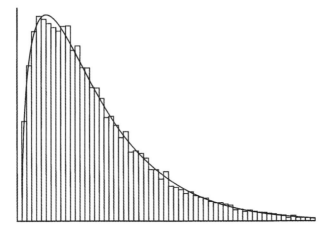

Figure 2.9 *Frequency distributions*
When a histogram is based on a large number of observations whose range is divided into fine intervals, the outline of the rectangles may take on the shape of a smooth curve. This curve is known as the frequency distribution of the variable that has been measured

The secret of constructing a useful histogram is the choice of intervals into which the range of measurements is divided. If the intervals are too narrow we end up with a picture similar to a bar chart, and if they are too wide we lose useful detail (fig 2.8). Getting the right balance is to some extent a matter of trial and error. Statistical packages for computers are programmed to make a sensible choice of intervals for histograms, but the user normally has the option to alter the specification if desired.

Frequency distributions

When a histogram is based on a large number of measurements it is possible to divide their range into relatively fine intervals, and the outline of the rectangles may then approximate to the form of a smooth curve (fig 2.9). This curve maps out the *frequency distribution* of the variable.

23

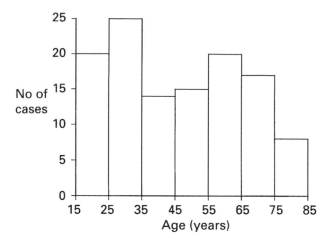

Figure 2.10 *Histogram showing the age distribution of 119 patients admitted to an oncology unit with Hodgkin's disease*
The distribution of patients is bimodal with peaks at age 25–34 and 55–64 years

The shape of the frequency distribution as plotted in a histogram can be characterised in several ways. One feature is the number of peaks that are observed. The distribution of blood pressures in figure 2.6 has a single peak or *mode* and is termed *unimodal*. On the other hand, the age distribution of patients admitted to an oncology unit with Hodgkin's disease, as shown in figure 2.10, is *bimodal* with two peaks.

Another feature is the symmetry of the distribution. The blood pressures in figure 2.6 are distributed in an approximately symmetrical fashion about a mode somewhere between 130 mm Hg and 139 mm Hg. In contrast, the survival periods of patients with colonic cancer illustrated in figure 2.11 have an asymmetrical or *skewed* distribution. The right-hand tail of the distribution is longer than the left, and we therefore say that it is skewed to the right or positively skewed. Conversely, where the left-hand tail of a unimodal distribution is longer than the right, the distribution is skewed to the left or negatively skewed. Note that in a symmetrical distribution the mean is equal to the median.

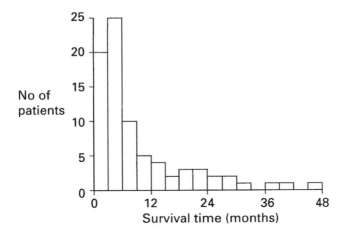

Figure 2.11 *Histogram showing survival periods from diagnosis in a series of patients with colonic cancer*

In addition, 21 patients were still alive after four years of follow-up. The distribution of survival times is skewed to the right—that is, it is asymmetrical with a longer right-hand than left-hand tail

The normal distribution

Certain shapes of frequency distribution occur frequently in nature (at least to a close approximation) and are given special names. One in particular, to which reference is often made, is the *normal distribution* (sometimes also known as the *Gaussian distribution*). This has a symmetrical bell shape (fig 2.12) that can be described by a mathematical equation. Sometimes the bell is tall and narrow, and sometimes it is more flattened, but whatever the dispersion of the data, approximately 95% of measurements lie within two standard deviations either side of the mean.

As well as allowing us to describe succinctly a commonly observed pattern of data, the concept of the normal distribution is important in the mathematics of statistical inference.

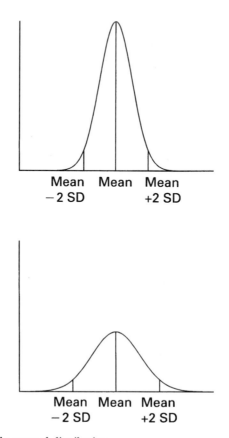

Figure 2.12 *The normal distribution*
This has a symmetrical bell-shape. The bell may be tall and narrow or more flattened, but whatever the dispersion of the data, approximately 95% of observations lie within two standard deviations (SD) either side of the mean

Questions

2.1 Which of the following could be summarised by a histogram?

(a) The distribution of a series of leukaemia patients according to HLA type.

(b) The weekly numbers of appendicectomies carried out in a surgical unit over a 12 month period.

(c) The serum concentrations of γ-glutamyl transferase in a series of alcoholic patients.

(d) The numbers of cardiac arrests experienced by each of a group of patients while on a coronary care unit.

2.2 Which of the following could be summarised by a bar chart?

(a) The numbers of filled teeth in a series of 5-year old children.

(b) The distribution of a series of women undergoing cervical smear testing according to whether the findings were normal, suspicious, or definitely abnormal.

(c) The distribution of peak flow measurements in a group of patients with chronic bronchitis.

(d) The activity of serum amylase in a series of patients presenting to hospital with acute abdominal pain.

2.3 Which of the following could be summarised by a mean and standard deviation?

(a) The numbers of hospital admissions required in a group of patients with inflammatory bowel disease followed over two years.

(b) The head circumferences of a sample of newborn babies measured in cm.

(c) The grades of hypertensive retinopathy in a group of patients receiving treatment for high blood pressure.

    (d) The annual amounts spent on drugs in 30 general practices.

2.4 Which of the following apply to a variable with a normal distribution?

    (a) Its distribution is skewed to the right.

    (b) Its distribution is unimodal.

    (c) Its mean is equal to its median.

3 Summarising bivariate and multivariate data

Bivariate data

Summaries of bivariate data provide information about the distribution and interrelation of two variables. Each of the variables may be nominal, ordinal, discrete quantitative, or continuous quantitative, so there are a total of 10 possible combinations:

nominal × nominal
nominal × ordinal
ordinal × ordinal
nominal × discrete quantitative
ordinal × discrete quantitative
discrete quantitative × discrete quantitative
nominal × continuous quantitative
ordinal × continuous quantitative
discrete quantitative × continuous quantitative
continuous quantitative × continuous quantitative

These will be considered in turn.

Both variables nominal

When both variables are nominal, it is often convenient to set out a numerical summary in the form of a *contingency table*. For example, table 3.1 shows the distribution of a series of stomach cancer patients according to their blood group and the histological type of the tumour. One variable (blood group) is represented by the columns of the table, and the other (histology) by the rows. The cells of the table show the counts of patients for each combination of

Table 3.1 A contingency table showing the distribution of a series of stomach cancer patients according to blood group and histology. Percentages are based on the total study sample of 490 patients as a denominator

Histology	Blood group				
	A	B	AB	O	Total
Intestinal type	127	72	32	95	326
	(26%)	(15%)	(7%)	(19%)	(67%)
Diffuse	80	25	11	48	164
	(16%)	(5%)	(2%)	(10%)	(33%)
Total	207	97	43	143	490
	(42%)	(20%)	(9%)	(29%)	(100%)

Table 3.2 Contingency table showing the proportions (%) of men in an epidemiological survey who reported back pain in the previous 12 months, according to employment status

Back pain in previous 12 months	Employment status	
	Employed (n = 1037)	Unemployed (n = 128)
Yes	37	45
No	63	55

The denominators on which the proportions are based are given at the head of each column. Because the back pain variable can only take one of two values, "yes" or "no," the second row of the table is redundant and could reasonably be omitted

blood group and histology, and as an option the *marginal totals* (the totals for each column and row) are also displayed. In this particular example there are four columns and two rows, but any number of each is permissible, depending on the numbers of categories into which the variables fall. A contingency table showing the distribution of the patients by sex and histology would have two rows and two columns.

As an alternative or in addition to frequency counts, the proportion of observations in each cell can be calculated. In table 3.1 the proportions are expressed as a fraction of all patients, but usually it is more informative to take the marginal totals of the columns or rows as the denominators. For example, table 3.2 gives the proportions of men in an epidemiological survey who reported back pain in the previous 12 months, according to whether they were in work or unemployed at the time of answering a

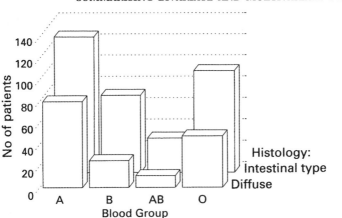

Figure 3.1 *A three-dimensional bar chart based on the data summarised in table 3.1*
This method of presentation is satisfactory provided that some bars do not get completely hidden behind others

questionnaire. In this case the proportions are based on the totals for each column. If, as here, proportions are quoted without giving the frequency count for each individual cell of the contingency table, it is usually helpful at least to indicate the total counts on which the proportions are based.

Because the variable "back pain in the past 12 months" as defined in this survey could take only two values—"yes" or "no"—the information in the second row of table 3.2 is really redundant. Once we know that 45% of unemployed men reported the symptom, it follows automatically that $100 - 45 = 55\%$ did not. Thus in this case it would be quite reasonable to omit the second row. However, if the variable had three categories (perhaps because some men could not remember whether they had had back symptoms and were thus classed as "don't know"), a one line summary giving the proportions of men reporting back pain would not convey all of the information. We would not know what proportions of men belonged to the "don't know" as opposed to the "no" category.

As with univariate data, spurious precision in the calculation of proportions should be avoided.

The information in table 3.1 can be represented graphically by a three dimensional bar chart (fig 3.1). This method works well

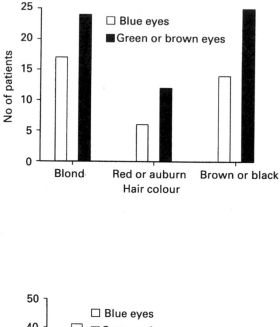

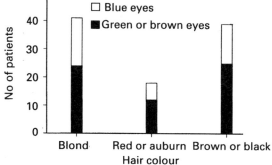

Figure 3.2 *Bar charts showing counts of patients with melanoma according to eye and hair colour. The two charts are alternative methods of presenting the data*

provided that some bars do not get completely hidden behind others; this will depend on the distribution of the data. If the problem does arise, it is better to show a series of bar charts side by side as in figure 3.2. The top part of figure 3.2 shows counts of melanoma patients according to their eye and hair colour. There is one bar chart for each category of hair colour, with the individual

32

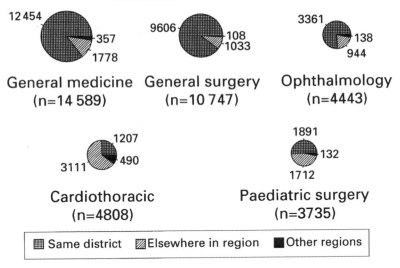

General medicine (n=14 589)

General surgery (n=10 747)

Ophthalmology (n=4443)

Cardiothoracic (n=4808)

Paediatric surgery (n=3735)

▦ Same district ▨ Elsewhere in region ■ Other regions

Figure 3.3 *Use of multiple pie charts to show the distribution of hospital admissions according to department and catchment population*

Each of the five departments is represented by a separate pie whose area corresponds to the total number of admissions by that department over a 12 month period. The pies are divided up to show the proportions of these admissions from different catchment populations

bars representing different colours of eyes. The bars are shaded to help clarify the eye colours to which they refer (colour coding would be better, but makes books more expensive). Alternatively, the bar charts could be combined, as in the lower figure where each bar represents a category of hair colour and is divided into segments corresponding to different eye colours. The height of the segment indicates the count of patients with the relevant combination of hair and eye colour.

Another way of displaying bivariate nominal data graphically uses multiple pie charts, as in figure 3.3. Each category of one variable (in this example "specialty") is represented by a separate pie, the area of which corresponds to the total number of hospital admissions for that specialty during a 12 month period. The pies are divided up to show the proportions of these admissions from different catchment populations. Again, colour coding would be an advantage.

33

Contingency table showing numbers of subjects

Grade of cataract	Pterygium	
	Absent	Present
0	189	7
I	270	7
II	236	8
III	218	6
IV	40	1

Barchart

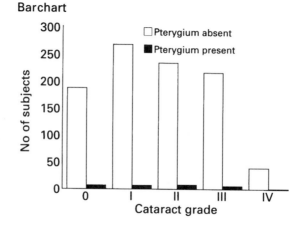

Figure 3.4 *Two methods of summarising the distribution of subjects in a survey of eye disease according to grade of cataract and presence or absence of pterygium in the right eye*

The ordering of cataract grades is respected in both methods of presentation

Each of these methods of graphical display has its advantages, and the choice between them is largely a matter of personal taste. You pick the one that you feel conveys the message most simply and clearly.

Table 3.3   Contingency table showing agreement between two doctors when asked to grade femoral neck bone mass independently in a series of 100 radiographs

Grade assigned by second doctor	Grade assigned by first doctor					
	1	2	3	4	5	6
1						
2		7		1		
3		1	24	9	1	
4			5	38	3	
5				1	9	1
6						

The grades of bone mass are set out in their natural order on both axes. Thus, the diagonal represents exact concordance between the two observers, and the further a pair of observations lies from the diagonal, the more the disagreement. Cells of the table with a zero count have in this case been left blank

One variable nominal and one variable ordinal or both variables ordinal

In this situation the methods of summary are similar to those used when both variables are nominal, but with the additional requirement that the categories of ordinal variables are presented in their natural order. For example, figure 3.4 shows the distribution of subjects in a survey of eye disease according to grade of cataract (an ordinal variable) and the presence or absence of pterygium (a nominal variable). The analysis was carried out because both diseases are suspected of being caused by exposure to ultraviolet radiation in sunlight. Note that the cataract grades are displayed in order from zero to four, both in the contingency table and in the bar chart.

Table 3.3 illustrates the level of agreement between two doctors when asked independently to grade femoral neck bone mass in a series of pelvic radiographs. The grading, which depends on the trabecular pattern of the bone, is according to an index devised by Singh. Here both variables are ordinal. The ranking of both is taken into account in the presentation, and with the data summarised in this way, the diagonal from the top left to the bottom right hand corner of the table represents exact concordance between the two observers. The further a pair of observations lies from this diagonal, the greater the disagreement.

Table 3.4 Contingency table showing case fatality in patients with myocardial infarction according to number of previous infarcts

No of previous infarcts	No of patients	Proportion (%) of cases fatal
0	35	20
1	25	28
2	9	22
3	5	40
4	2	50
All patients	76	25

The row totals on which the proportions are based are given in the central column. As all cases are classed either as "fatal" or "not fatal" (there are no "unknowns"), there is no need for a column to show the proportions of cases that were not fatal

One variable nominal or ordinal and one variable discrete quantitative

If the quantitative variable does not take too many values (up to five or six, say), one option is to summarise the data in the form of a contingency table as in table 3.4. Often, however, a better approach is to derive summary measures of central tendency and dispersion for the quantitative variable across each category of the nominal or ordinal variable. These can then be displayed in tabular form or graphically. Thus, figure 3.5 shows two ways of summarising the frequency of admissions to a district general hospital for attempted suicide on different days of the week over the course of a year. Note that with either method, the days of the week are in their proper sequence.

Both variables discrete quantitative

If neither variable takes too many values, a contingency table may again be helpful. For example, table 3.5 shows the number of units of blood transfused in patients with haematemesis and melaena according to the occurrence of rebleeding episodes while they were in hospital.

36

Day of week	No of admissions		
	Mean	Median	Range
Monday	1·4	1·0	0–5
Tuesday	1·6	1·0	0–5
Wednesday	2·0	2·0	0–10
Thursday	1·8	1·5	0–7
Friday	1·9	2·0	0–6
Saturday	1·4	1·0	0–4
Sunday	1·6	2·0	0–4

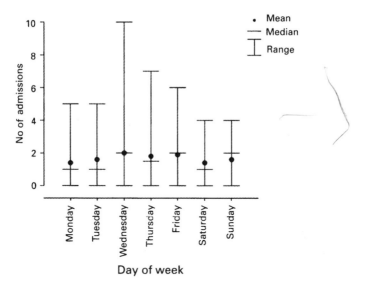

Figure 3.5 *Two methods of summarising the frequency of admissions to a district general hospital for attempted suicide on different days of the week over the course of a year*

Table 3.5 Contingency table showing number of units of blood transfused in patients with haematemesis and melaena according to the occurrence of rebleeding episodes while in hospital

Number of units of blood transfused	Number of episodes of rebleeding			
	0	1	2	Total
0	210	0	0	210
2	18	0	0	18
4	99	4	0	103
6	55	51	0	106
8	10	35	8	53
10	0	8	22	30
Total	392	98	30	520

Where the number of values taken by a variable is larger, it may be preferable to calculate univariate summary statistics for it across the values of the other variable and then display them either in tabular or graphical form. Thus, figure 3.6 shows how the number of episodes of reduced peak flow in a group of children over a 12 month period related to the dose of methacholine which produced a reduction of at least 20% in FEV_1 (forced expiratory volume in one second) in a bronchial challenge test. This is the provocative dose (PD_{20}). The methacholine was given in incremental doses, stopping when the FEV_1 had fallen by 20% from baseline. Because there were only three children with a PD_{20} of 0·05 and two with a PD_{20} of 0·2, it might be better to group together those with a $PD_{20} \leq 0·2$ µmol methacholine, as in figure 3.6(c), putting a break in the horizontal axis to make clear that they have been treated differently.

One variable nominal, ordinal or discrete quantitative, and one variable continuous quantitative

A commonly used method of summary is to calculate measures of central tendency and dispersion for the continuous variable across the values of the other variable. These can then be shown

38

SUMMARISING BIVARIATE AND MULTIVARIATE DATA

(a) Tabular summary

PD$_{20}$ (μmol methacholine)	No of children	No of episodes Median	Range
0·05	3	3	0–5
0·1	8	3	1–8
0·2	2	4	3–5
0·4	7	2	0–6
0·8	5	3	1–4
1·6	8	4·5	2–8
3·2	10	3	1–8
6·4	13	3	1–8

(b) Graphical summary

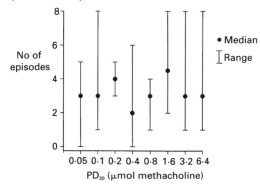

(c) Graphical summary (alternative method)

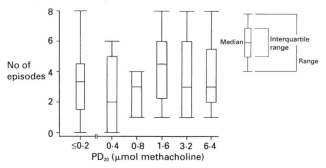

Figure 3.6 *Three methods of summarising the relation of the number of episodes of reduced peak flow in a group of children over 12 months to PD$_{20}$ on methacholine challenge*

For ease of presentation, PD$_{20}$ in the graphs is plotted on a logarithmic scale (see page 43). The second graph shows interquartile ranges as well as medians and ranges

39

(a) *Tabular representation*

Time	Blood glucose (mmol/l)	
(minutes)	Mean	Standard deviation
0	5.6	0.5
30	8.7	0.9
120	6.0	1.2

(b) **Graphical representation of means and standard deviations**

(c) *Dot plot*

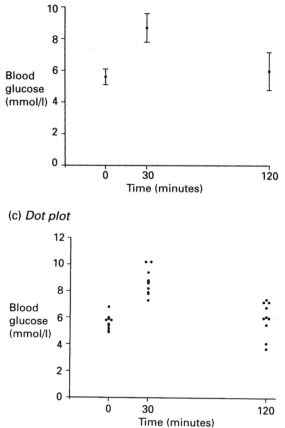

Figure 3.7 *Four methods of summarising the results of 10 oral glucose tolerance tests (continued)*

(d) *Dots linked for each patient*

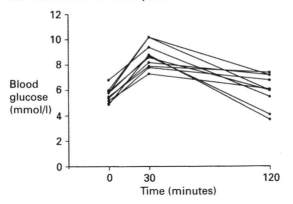

Figure 3.7 *Four methods of summarising the results of 10 oral glucose tolerance tests*

either in tabular or in graphical form. Figure 3.7 shows two ways ((a) and (b)) of illustrating the distribution of blood glucose concentrations recorded at different intervals after initial loading in a series of oral glucose tolerance tests. Sampling was carried out at 0, 30, and 120 minutes.

A more complete graphical description is provided by a "dot plot", in which values of the nominal, ordinal, or discrete quantitative variable are represented on one axis (in order and to scale if appropriate) and the continuous variable is displayed on the other axis. Each observation is then marked as a dot, as in figure 3.7(c). Where two or more observations coincide, their dots can be plotted alongside each other. In this example, two patients had glucose levels of 7·2 mmol/l at 120 minutes.

A limitation of the dot plot shown here is that it does not indicate which dots belong to which patients. If it were important to convey this information, the three dots for each patient could be joined by lines, as in figure 3.7(d). It now becomes clear that those with high glucose at 30 minutes tended also to have high values at 120 minutes. With a large number of patients, however, a plot of this type could get rather messy.

41

(a) *When IgE is plotted on a linear scale most of the dots are clustered near the baseline, making them difficult to distinguish.*

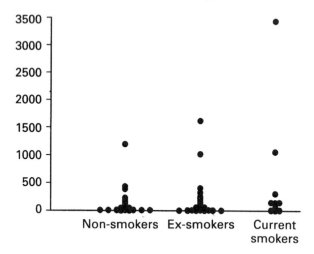

(b) *The picture becomes clearer when IgE is plotted on a logarithmic scale.*

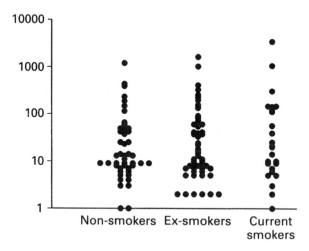

Figure 3.8 *Dot plots showing serum immunoglobulin E (IgE) in IU/ml according to smoking habits in a sample of elderly men and women*

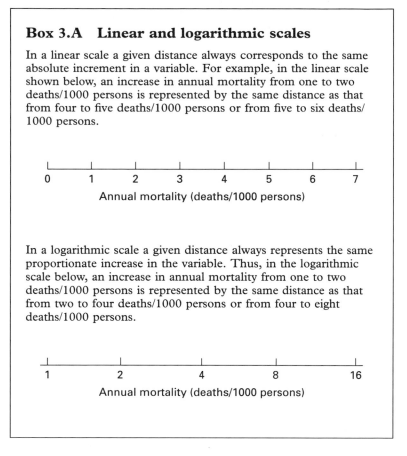

Box 3.A   Linear and logarithmic scales

In a linear scale a given distance always corresponds to the same absolute increment in a variable. For example, in the linear scale shown below, an increase in annual mortality from one to two deaths/1000 persons is represented by the same distance as that from four to five deaths/1000 persons or from five to six deaths/1000 persons.

```
L_____L_____L_____L_____L_____L_____L_____L
0           1           2           3           4           5           6           7
```
Annual mortality (deaths/1000 persons)

In a logarithmic scale a given distance always represents the same proportionate increase in the variable. Thus, in the logarithmic scale below, an increase in annual mortality from one to two deaths/1000 persons is represented by the same distance as that from two to four deaths/1000 persons or from four to eight deaths/1000 persons.

```
_|_____|_____|_____|_____|_
1                     2                     4                     8                    16
```
Annual mortality (deaths/1000 persons)

Sometimes the continuous variable has a highly skewed distribution. For example, the dot plot in figure 3.8(a) shows serum levels of immunoglobulin E in non-smokers, ex-smokers, and current smokers. Most of the dots are clustered near the baseline (zero), making them difficult to distinguish. In this situation the picture may be made clearer by plotting the continuous variable on a *logarithmic scale*, as in figure 3.8(b). Normally we use a *linear scale* in which a given distance always corresponds to the same absolute increment in the variable. In a logarithmic scale a given distance always corresponds to the same proportionate increase in the variable (box 3.A). The effect of using a logarithmic scale is

43

to compress the upper end of a range relative to the lower end. Differences between high values look less impressive. Thus when reading graphs it is important always to check the type of scale. Note also that a logarithmic scale can never get down to zero. For example, suppose that we are summarising weights and that a distance of 5 mm on our scale corresponds to a doubling of weight. If we start at the point on the scale representing 1 g and go down 5 mm we will get to a value of 0·5 g. Another 5 mm down will take us to 0·25 g. But no matter how long we continue in this way, we will never reach a weight of zero. It follows that if a variable sometimes takes a value of zero, or can take both positive and negative values, then it cannot be displayed on a logarithmic scale.

Both variables continuous quantitative

The relation between two continuous variables can be displayed graphically as a *scatter plot*. One variable is represented on the horizontal axis and the other on the vertical axis. Each pair of measurements is then represented as a dot. For example, figure 3.9 illustrates the relation between mortality rates from chronic bronchitis in 212 local authority areas of England and Wales during 1968–78 and infant mortality from respiratory disease in the same areas some 50 years earlier.

Conventionally, if one variable can be considered to depend on or be caused by the other, it is called the *dependent variable* and is drawn on the vertical axis. The other variable is termed the *independent variable* and is shown on the horizontal axis. In figure 3.9 it is more natural to think of mortality from chronic bronchitis in 1968–78 depending on earlier patterns of infant mortality than the other way round.

If it makes the presentation clearer, one or both variables may be plotted on a logarithmic scale.

The most common form of numerical summary for bivariate continuous data is the *correlation coefficient*. This is a measure of the extent to which the points in a scatter plot lie on a straight line. It is calculated from the paired measurements according to a set formula or rule (normally this is done by a computer program in a statistical package) and can take values between -1 and $+1$. A negative correlation coefficient implies that the points fit best to a straight line sloping down from left to right, and a value of -1

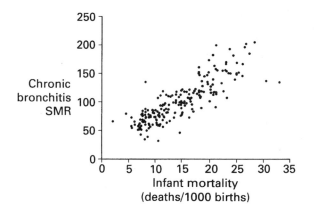

Figure 3.9 *Scatter plot illustrating the relation between mortality from chronic bronchitis at ages 35–74 in 212 local authority areas of England and Wales during 1968–78 and infant mortality from respiratory disease in the same areas during 1921–25*

Mortality from chronic bronchitis is expressed in terms of a standardised mortality ratio (SMR) to take account of possible differences in the age distribution of the populations under examination. The striking relation between the two sets of mortality rates suggests that causes of respiratory infection in infancy may also predispose to later chronic obstructive airways disease

means that the points lie perfectly on such a line (fig 3.10). A positive coefficient implies that the best fitting straight line slopes up from left to right, and a value of +1 means that the points lie perfectly on a line sloping in this way. The closer the correlation coefficient to zero, the less well the points fit to a straight line.

Note that a correlation coefficient of zero does not mean that two variables are not related—only that they do not have a straight line relationship. Thus in figure 3.10(f) the independent variable seems to determine the dependent variable precisely, but because the relationship is not *linear* the correlation coefficient may be close to zero.

45

(a)

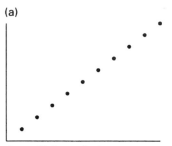

A coefficient of +1 means a
perfect fit to a straight line
rising from left to right

(b)

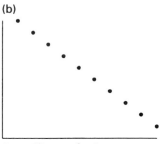

A coefficent of −1 means a
perfect fit to a straight line
sloping down from left to right

(c)

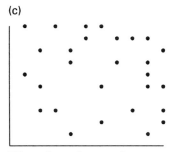

When the points on the scatter
plot show a poor fit to a straight
line, the correlation coefficient
is close to zero

(d)

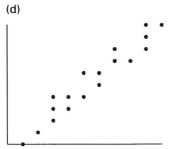

Here the points show an
imperfect fit to a straight line
rising from left to right. The
correlation coefficient is +0·96

(e)

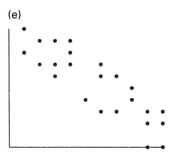

A rather poorer fit to a straight
line than (d) and sloping down
from left to right. The coefficient
is −0·87

(f)

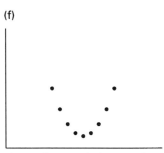

A non-linear relation can have a
correlation coefficient close to
zero even if it is very exact

Figure 3.10 *Correlation coefficients*

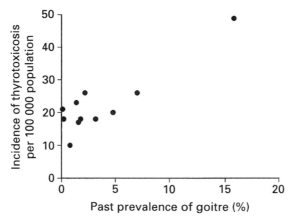

Figure 3.11 *A scatter plot showing the correlation of incidence of thyrotoxicosis and past prevalence of goitre in 11 British towns*
One outlying town has an unusually high rate of both thyrotoxicosis and goitre. Such outliers have a strong influence on correlation coefficients. In this instance, exclusion of the outlier reduces the correlation coefficient from 0·89 to 0·47

It is important to note that correlation coefficients can be strongly influenced by a few outlying points on the scatter plot. In figure 3.11, which shows the relation of thyrotoxicosis incidence to the past prevalence of goitre in 11 British towns, exclusion of the outlying point reduces the correlation coefficient from 0·89 to 0·47. For this reason, when analysing bivariate continuous data it is wise to examine scatter plots as well as calculating correlation coefficients.

The other common method of summarising bivariate continuous data is by means of a *regression line*. This is the straight line that best fits the points on a scatter plot, and like the correlation coefficient it is derived according to set rules (usually by means of a program in a statistical package). It can be superimposed on the scatter plot, as in figure 3.12, or expressed in terms of an equation. For example, the regression line in figure 3.12 is such that, on average, an increase in infant mortality from bronchitis and pneumonia of 10 deaths per 1000 births is associated with an increase of 52 in the standardised mortality ratio (SMR) for chronic bronchitis.

47

(a) A regression line is the straight line which best fits the points on a scatter plot. The figure below shows a regression line superimposed on the scatter plot from fig 3.9

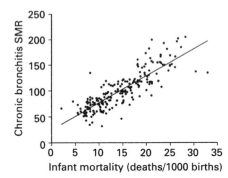

The use of a regression line is in predicting values of the dependent variable from the independent variable. For example, from the regression line above we would predict the SMR from chronic bronchitis in an area to be:

25 + (5·2 × its infant mortality rate from bronchitis and pneumonia.)

The prediction is only valid within the range of data from which it has been derived. It should not be used for extrapolation (as opposed to interpolation).

(b) A regression line can be calculated even when the data show minimal tendency to a linear relationship:

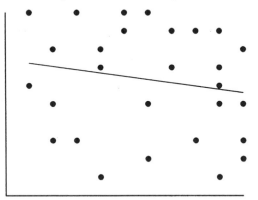

However, in this case the regression line has little meaning.

Figure 3.12 *Regression lines*

A regression line is the straight line which best fits the data, but unlike the correlation coefficient, it does not indicate how good the fit is. A regression line can be calculated even when the data show minimal tendency to a linear relationship. In this case, however, the regression line has little meaning. The use of the regression line is in predicting values of the dependent variable from the independent variable. For example, from the regression line in figure 3.12(a) it can be predicted that an infant mortality rate from bronchitis and pneumonia of 20 deaths per 1000 births will be associated with an SMR for chronic bronchitis of 129. Such predictions are valid only within the range of the data. The regression line in figure 3.12(a) could not validly be used to predict the chronic bronchitis SMR associated with an infant mortality from respiratory disease of 40 deaths per 1000 births. Clearly, when the correlation coefficient is close to zero, as in figure 3.12(b), one can have little confidence in predictions based on a regression line. Techniques of statistical inference based on regression are discussed in chapter 8.

Multivariate data

When data sets comprise more than two interrelated variables, summary becomes more difficult. The best approach is often to start by looking at each variable separately in univariate analyses and then proceed to examine them in pairs. For example, in the multivariate set of data on births that was discussed in chapter 1, one might first summarise the distribution of each individual variable and then analyse the relation of birth weight to each of sex, social class, and number of previous pregnancies. Exploration in this way gives a feel for the structure of the data and allows important features to be characterised. The interrelationship of multiple variables may be further summarised by techniques of statistical modelling, but this is more often carried out in the context of statistical inference than for simple description (see chapter 8).

Guiding principles

The description of methods of summarising data that has been presented here and in chapter 2 is not comprehensive, but it covers the techniques that are most often encountered in medical practice. The first step in an analysis is to identify the types of data under consideration. Various approaches are then possible for each type of data, and the choice is partly a matter of personal preference. The guiding principle should be to abstract and convey the important messages of the data in the simplest and clearest way possible. Graphs are often better than tables when the need is to provide a summary message that can be assimilated rapidly. On the other hand, tables usually give more precise information and may allow readers to carry out further calculations on the data if they wish. Tables and graphs should be adequately labelled, especially in written reports. The need for simplicity applies particularly to visual aids for oral presentations. Too often speakers succumb to temptation and try to include more information in a slide than can reasonably be assimilated by their audience.

Questions

3.1 What methods could be used to summarise the following?

(a) The presence or absence of cutaneous warts in groups of men from four different occupational groups.

(b) The relation between length of stay in an intensive care unit (measured in days) and Glasgow coma score (measured on an ordinal scale from 0 to 15) on admission in a series of patients.

(c) The relation between APGAR score at birth (measured on an ordinal scale from 0 to 10) and IQ at age 7 years in a sample of children born on a maternity unit.

(d) The presence or absence of Parkinson's disease in relation to smoking habit (classed as non-smoker, ex-smoker, or current smoker) in a survey of elderly people.

(e) The case fatality of a series of children with bacterial meningitis according to the day of the week on which they were admitted to hospital.

(f) The relation of birth weight to fasting blood glucose concentration at age 50 years in a sample of men born at the same hospital during the 1940s.

(g) The agreement between two surgeons in classifying inguinal hernias as direct or indirect on clinical examination.

4 Probability

Chapters 2 and 3 have dealt with techniques for summarising data. Sometimes our interest extends no further than the data set that is being summarised. Thus, in a parliamentary election the distribution of votes cast on the day directly determines the outcome of interest—who is elected and who loses their deposit. This contrasts with an opinion poll, where our primary concern is not the voting preference of the sample of people interviewed, but that of the electorate more generally. We hope that the distribution of preferences in the interviewees tells us something about this, but there is always a possibility that the people selected for interview are in some way atypical.

The same distinction can be drawn in medical practice. A consultant wishing to justify a short term increase in manpower for his outpatient clinic needs information about the patients on his waiting list. He might summarise this in terms of the mean time since referral of those currently waiting for a first appointment, or by the proportion who have been waiting for more than six months. Whether the current state of affairs is atypical (for example, because of an unusual spate of referrals or sickness absence in staff) is irrelevant to the short term decision. If patients have been waiting too long then something needs to be done. The patients studied form the total population of interest.

On the other hand, the observation of reduced mortality in patients with myocardial infarction who are given a thrombolytic drug as part of a clinical trial is important only for what it can tell us about the value of the drug more generally (unless we happen to be one of the patients in the trial). This will depend on how well the findings in the sample of patients studied represent the wider state of affairs.

Samples may be unrepresentative because of the way in which they have been selected. For example, an opinion poll carried out by approaching people on the street and asking them for their views would tend to exclude people who do not get out and about—perhaps because they are tied up at work or because they are disabled. If the opinions of such men and women are different from those of people who walk around town then the findings of the survey are unlikely to reflect reliably the views of the total population. Similarly, a study of alcohol consumption in general practice patients could be misleading if the heaviest drinkers declined to participate. Where a sample is atypical of the larger population which it is intended to represent because of the way in which it has been chosen, we say that it is *biased*.

In addition, even if there is no systematic deficiency in its method of selection, a sample may be unrepresentative by chance. If I throw a die twice, the outcome will not necessarily be the same on both occasions. In fact, most times I would expect to throw different numbers. (If you have ever waited for a double to start a board game you will be well aware of this.) In the same way, two clinical trials with identical designs would not be expected to produce identical results. Differences will occur just by chance. The process of drawing conclusions from samples about wider populations while taking into account possible chance effects is known as *statistical inference*.

The principles of statistical inference will be described in chapters 5 to 8, but first we need a method of quantifying chance. This is achieved using a measure called *probability*. As I will show, the concept of probability is relevant not only to statistical inference but also to other aspects of medical practice.

What is chance?

Suppose that I toss a coin. In theory, if I knew all of the relevant physical factors, including the mass of the coin, its diameter and thickness, the exact forces setting it in motion, the viscosity of the air, the height of the surface onto which the coin will fall, and the shape and plasticity of this surface, I might be able to predict whether it will come down heads or tails. In practice, however, these cannot be known with sufficient accuracy or detail. Thus, in advance the outcome will always be uncertain—a matter of chance.

In the same way, I cannot predict with certainty whether an apparently healthy patient attending my clinic is going in the future to develop lung cancer. Certain influences make this outcome more or less likely (for example, his smoking habits), but it will depend upon a myriad of circumstances, many of them operating at a molecular level, about which I will never have adequate information. Whether the patient goes on to develop lung cancer is again a matter of chance.

Probability

Although I cannot reliably predict the outcome of an individual coin toss, I do know that if I toss a coin a large number of times it will tend to come down heads on half the tosses. The reasons for this must lie in the way that the many factors that determine the result of a single coin toss interact with each other. The practical importance is that it offers a way of quantifying the chance of throwing heads. If on repeated coin tossing half of all tosses result in heads, I can say that the probability of obtaining heads in a single toss is 50% or 0·5.*

Similarly, if I know from previous studies that 6% of men with the same age and smoking habits as my clinic patient will go on to develop lung cancer, I can say that the probability of my patient getting lung cancer is 6% or 0·06.

When they are defined in this way, we can see that probabilities are numbers in the range from zero to one. A probability of zero means that the outcome will never happen. A probability of one means that it will definitely occur. The closer the probability to one, the more likely the outcome.

In medical practice we often have to deal with uncertainties, and many of these can be quantified by probabilities. One application lies in the description of prognosis. Patients and their families regularly ask what are the chances that an operation will be successful or that a treatment will lead to cure, and the answer is often in the form of a probability. For example, we might tell the parents of a baby newly diagnosed as having leukaemia that with current treatment there is a 30% chance of a cure.

Sometimes the probabilities we give are rough guesses based on our personal clinical experience, but in other cases they may derive from formal research. For example, a systematic follow up study

---

* In this and the chapters that follow, percentages and decimals are used interchangeably.

of adults presenting with a first epileptic fit collected information about the occurrence of further fits in the same patients over the next few years. This helps us to estimate the probability that a person with a first seizure will go on to have more fits, an important consideration in deciding whether he or she should be allowed to continue driving a car.

Of course, when quantifying prognosis in this way it is important to take into account as far as possible those factors that are likely to have a major influence on the course of an illness. Thus, if the staging of a tumour is known and is a crucial determinant of outcome, we should base our prognosis and any probabilities that we quote on experience relating specifically to that tumour stage.

Another application of probabilities relates to the diagnostic process. When a patient presents with a complaint we assess the chances of different underlying diagnoses and plan our investigation or treatment accordingly. For example, a general practitioner confronted by a child with a sore throat would assess the probability of a bacterial cause, taking into account which upper respiratory infections were prevalent in the community at the time and any special diagnostic features of the case. Depending on this evaluation the doctor might prescribe an antibiotic, take a throat swab, or treat the symptoms and review the child if there was no improvement over the next few days. If a throat swab were taken and proved negative on bacterial culture, this would lead the doctor to modify his or her assessment of the probability of bacterial infection.

In experimental trials where computers have been used to assist diagnosis, the programs have been based on numerical calculations of probability, but normally the assessment of the chances of different diagnosis is informal and more qualitative. Nevertheless, an understanding of probability helps to clarify the process. Also, it offers a way of quantifying the value of different diagnostic tests and procedures.

Sensitivity, specificity, and predictive value

Few clinical investigations are completely reliable, and errors can occur in both directions. Some patients may be incorrectly classified as having a disease (false positive diagnoses), while others

Box 4.A Evaluation of mammography in the diagnosis of breast cancer

Outcomes in a series of 1500 women investigated by mammography

Result of mammography	Histologically proven tumour within six months of mammography		Total
	Yes	No	
Positive	9	59	68
Negative	7	1425	1432
Total	16	1484	1500

The sensitivity of mammography is the probability that it will correctly diagnose a true case, and is given by 9/16 = 56%

The specificity of mammography is the probability that it will correctly classify a non-case, and is given by 1425/1484 = 96%

The predictive value of mammography is the probability that a woman with a positive result really has a tumour, and is given by 9/68 = 13%

who are genuine cases may be missed (false negative diagnoses). If correct diagnoses can eventually be established then the accuracy of a test can be evaluated. For example, box 4.A shows the accuracy of mammography in the diagnosis of breast cancer, assessed according to whether a histologically proven tumour was found at some stage during the six months after the test. (It is assumed here that histology provides a valid guide as to whether a cancer is really present, although in practice histology too might be misleading.) Of 1500 women in the study, 16 turned out to have breast cancer, and nine of these had been correctly diagnosed on mammography. The proportion of cases correctly diagnosed by a test is known as its *sensitivity*. Put another way, the sensitivity of a test is the probability that it will correctly diagnose a case.

A total of 1484 women did not have breast cancer, and 1425 of these were correctly classified as cancer-free on mammography. The proportion of non-cases correctly classified by a test is termed its *specificity*. In other words, specificity represents the probability that a non-case will be correctly classified.

The requirements of a test in terms of sensitivity and specificity depend on the use to which it is to be put. For a screening exercise that is to be followed by more detailed investigation of people with positive tests (for example, cervical smear testing in which positive results are followed up by cone biopsy), the emphasis is usually on sensitivity—on ensuring that cases are not missed. On the other hand, when a positive diagnosis on a test will lead directly to a major intervention such as colectomy or mastectomy, high specificity is essential. If the test lacks specificity, a substantial number of people may receive unnecessary and injurious treatment.

The characteristic of a test that is of most relevance in the management of an individual patient is its *predictive value*—the probability that disease is really present when the test is positive. In box 4.A, 13% of women with positive mammograms actually had breast cancer.

The predictive value of a test depends on the prevalence of disease in the population of patients to whom it is applied. Consider the example of sputum cytology as an investigation for bronchial carcinoma. Let us suppose that the test has a sensitivity of 40% and a specificity of 99%.

The first example in box 4.B shows the expected outcome if we apply the test in a sample of 1000 patients presenting to hospital with haemoptysis, 80% of whom have bronchial carcinoma. From the known sensitivity and specificity we would expect 320 of the 800 cases to test positive and 198 of the 200 non-cases to test negative. Altogether, therefore, we would have 322 patients with positive results, of whom 320 would really have lung cancer. It follows that the predictive value would be 320/322 = 99%.

By the same reasoning, the expected outcome if the test were used to screen 10 000 apparently healthy smokers with a lung cancer prevalence of 1% would be as in the second example in box 4.B. In this case the predictive value of 29% is much lower. Fewer than one third of the people with positive results would actually have lung cancer.

It is important for doctors to be aware that the predictive value of a test varies according to the circumstances of its use. Otherwise, they may manage patients inappropriately.

Box 4.B   **Application of sputum cytology as an investigation for bronchial carcinoma in two populations of patients**

It is assumed that the test has a sensitivity of 40% and specificity of 99%

(a) Expected outcome in 1000 patients presenting to hospital with haemoptysis of whom 80% have bronchial carcinoma

Sputum cytology	Bronchial carcinoma		Total
	Present	Absent	
Positive	320	2	322
Negative	480	198	678
Total	800	200	1000

Predictive value = 320/322 = 99%

(b) Expected outcome in 10 000 apparently healthy smokers with a lung cancer prevalence of 1%

Sputum cytology	Bronchial carcinoma		Total
	Present	Absent	
Positive	40	99	139
Negative	60	9801	9861
Total	100	9900	10 000

Predictive value = 40/139 = 29%

Combining probabilities

Either of two events

Where two outcomes are mutually exclusive, the probability that one or the other will occur is calculated by adding their individual probabilities. For example, if a baby has a 0·04% chance of being homozygous for the sickle cell gene and a 3·92% chance of being

58

a heterozygote, then the probability that it carries the gene either as a homozygote or as a heterozygote is $0.04 + 3.92 = 3.96\%$. Note that this rule for adding probabilities applies only when the outcomes are mutually exclusive. The probability that a baby carries genes for sickle cell disease and/or beta thalassaemia is not the probability that it carries the sickle cell gene plus the probability that it carries the beta thalassaemia gene. Rather, we must subtract from this sum the probability that the baby carries both the sickle cell and the beta thalassaemia genes. In general, for two outcomes A and B,

Probability of A or B = Probability of A + Probability of B
− Probability of both A and B

If A and B are mutually exclusive then they cannot both occur, and the probability of both A and B is therefore zero.

Both of two events

The probability that both of two events occur can be calculated from their separate probabilities if they are independent—if the occurrence of one event does not make the other more or less likely. In this case, the probability of both events occurring is obtained by multiplying their individual probabilities. This principle has important applications in medical genetics.

Suppose that a couple, both apparently healthy, have a child with cystic fibrosis. If they have another baby, what is the probability that this child too will have the disease? Cystic fibrosis is an autosomal recessive disorder. Each of us carries two copies of the relevant gene, one inherited from our father and one from our mother. The disease is manifest if both of these genes are defective. If a parent has a single defective gene (is a heterozygote) there is a 50% chance that the defective gene will be passed on to any son or daughter and a 50% chance that the child will receive the normal gene.

The parents in this example must be heterozygotes since they do not themselves have cystic fibrosis, but each must have passed on a defective gene to their child. Therefore if they have a second baby, there is a 50% chance that the gene transmitted from the father will be defective, and a 50% chance that the mother will

59

pass on a defective gene. From empirical observation we know that the transmission of genes from mother and father is independent. Getting a defective gene from the father makes no difference to the probability of being given a defective gene by the mother. It follows that the probability that the second child will have cystic fibrosis (because it has inherited a defective gene from both its father and its mother) is the probability of getting a defective gene from the father (0·5) multiplied by the probability of getting a defective gene from the mother (0·5). This comes to 0·25.

This is a very simple example, and clinical geneticists often have to advise on much more complex problems, but their calculations are guided by the basic rules for combining probabilities.

The other major application of probabilities in medicine is in statistical inference. This will be described in the chapters that follow.

Questions

4.1 Adult polycystic disease is autosomal dominant in inheritance. The disease occurs if a defective gene is inherited from either the mother or the father or from both parents. What is the probability that a man has polycystic disease if his sister has the disorder and his brother and father do not?

4.2 Surgeons were shown in one study to diagnose appendicitis correctly in patients with acute abdomen with sensitivity 88% and specificity 86%. Assuming that this is standard, what would be the predictive value of a surgeon's diagnosis of appendicitis in a sample of patients with acute abdomen, 25% of whom actually had the disorder?

4.3 The sensitivity and specificity of defined ECG criteria in the diagnosis of myocardial infarction are 80% and 50% respectively, while for criteria based on levels of cardiac enzymes the sensitivity and specificity are each 65%. Assuming that given the disease status of the patient, the results of the two tests are independent (in other words, among true cases of myocardial infarction a positive ECG does not make enzymes any more or less likely to be positive, and among non-cases a negative ECG does not make enzymes any more or less likely to be negative),

(a) What is the probability that a true case will be positive on both tests?

(b) What is the probability that a true case will be positive for either one or both tests?

(c) What is the probability that a non-case will be negative for both tests?

(d) What is the probability that a non-case will be negative for either one or both tests?

(e) If we took as our diagnostic criterion that both ECG and enzymes should be positive, what would be the sensitivity and specificity?

(f) If we took as our diagnostic criterion that either one or both of ECG and enzymes should be positive, what would be the sensitivity and specificity?

5 Hypothesis testing

Statistical inference is concerned with the uncertainties that arise when generalising from observations made in samples. Suppose, for example, that we carry out a laboratory experiment to test the chronic toxicity of a new drug, and we find that six out of 20 rats receiving the highest dose of the drug develop liver tumours as compared with only three out of 20 control animals. How sure can we be that this represents a genuine carcinogenic effect of the drug, and that repeat experiments with the same design would not show excesses of liver tumours in the controls as often as in the treated rats? Two approaches are commonly used to address such uncertainty. Hypothesis testing, which was the first of the methods to be developed, will be described in this chapter. Chapter 6 will describe the second technique, which is based on estimation with confidence intervals.

Populations and samples

Underlying all statistical inference, whether by hypothesis testing or by estimation with confidence intervals, is the notion that the available data relate to a *sample* and that this sample is derived from a larger *population* about which conclusions are to be drawn. The population of interest may be explicitly defined. For example, the sample of voters questioned in an opinion poll is selected from the electorate as a whole and is intended to provide information about the voting preferences of that larger population. More often, however, the population is hypothetical. Thus the sample of rats in a study of carcinogenicity is viewed as coming from a larger population of similar rats that might in theory be investigated in the same way. From observations in the sample we aim to draw conclusions about what would be found if the total population of rats were studied.

The mathematical theory underlying statistical inference generally assumes that the populations from which samples derive are extremely large. This is reasonable in most circumstances encountered in practice.

The logic behind hypothesis testing

Suppose that we are given a coin and are asked to find out whether it is a "fair" coin—whether it is equally likely to come down heads or tails when it is tossed. The obvious way to investigate this question is to toss the coin a few times and see what happens. If we tossed the coin three times and it came down heads on each occasion, we would not be terribly surprised. It quite often happens that a cricket or football captain wins the toss on three occasions in a row. However, if we then tossed the coin a further seven times and again got heads every time, we might begin to suspect something peculiar.

It would be nice if we could calculate a probability that the coin is fair, but with probability defined as in chapter 4, this is not possible. Our coin is not selected from a set of coins, known proportions of which are fair or unfair. The only information available to us is the outcome of the sample of coin tosses that we have carried out.

We can, however, turn the problem round and calculate what would be the probability of obtaining the outcome that we have observed if in fact the coin were fair. If the coin were fair, then in the hypothetical population of all tosses that could be made with it, half would be heads and half would be tails. Put another way, the probability that any single toss would come out heads is 0·5. Successive tosses of the same coin are independent. (The popular belief that if there has been a sequence of heads then tails is more likely next time by "the law of averages" is misguided.) It follows that the probability of three heads in a row is

$$0·5 \times 0·5 \times 0·5 = 0·125$$

Similarly, the probability of three tails in succession is 0·125. Throwing three successive heads and throwing three successive tails are mutually exclusive outcomes. Therefore the probability of obtaining three heads in a row *or* three tails in a row is

$$0.125 + 0.125 = 0.25$$

This accords with our intuition that three tosses in a row all the same is not terribly surprising. It can be expected to happen 25% of the time when we carry out three tosses with a fair coin.

If we toss a coin 10 times, the probability of getting 10 heads is

$$0.5 \times 0.5 \times 0.5 \times 0.5 \times 0.5 \times 0.5 \times 0.5 \times 0.5 \times 0.5 \times 0.5 = 0.00098$$

This is also the probability of obtaining 10 tails, and the probability of getting 10 tosses all the same (heads or tails) is therefore

$$0.00098 + 0.00098 = 0.00196$$

Again our intuitive judgment is supported. A sequence of 10 tosses all the same can happen with a fair coin, but it would occur on fewer than one in 500 occasions (0.00196 is less than $0.002 = 1/500$). Given that it is so improbable, we might feel inclined to reject the assumption of a fair coin as incorrect, and adopt the alternative view that the coin is unfair.

A parallel argument can be developed in the context of medical research. Suppose that we wish to investigate whether a new drug treatment for peptic ulcer is effective. Again, we might attempt to answer this question by conducting an experiment. We could set up a clinical trial in which a sample of patients with peptic ulcer was allocated to treatment either with the new drug or with a pharmacologically inactive placebo, and then compare the rate of healing (perhaps assessed by endoscopy) at a specified interval after starting treatment.

Suppose further that 60 out of 100 patients receiving the new drug are healed as compared with 30 out of 100 patients given placebo. As with the coin, it would be nice if we could calculate a probability that the drug is superior to placebo, but this does not make sense given the way in which probability has been defined. There is no set of "worlds" in a proportion of which the drug is effective while in the remainder it is no better than placebo. All

64

we have is our one "world" and the findings in our sample of 200 patients.

Again, a solution is found by turning the problem around. We can think of our sample of 200 patients as coming from an extremely large population of ulcer patients who could, in theory at least, be treated with drug or placebo. Let us assume that the drug is ineffective. If this is the case, the proportion of patients in our large population that would be healed while being given the drug would be the same as in patients receiving placebo. In other words, the probability of an individual patient receiving the drug being healed would be the same as that of an individual being given placebo.

In our sample of 200 patients the overall healing rate was

$$\frac{(60+30)}{(100+100)} = 45\%.$$

Assuming an underlying 45% probability of healing in the source population of ulcer patients, whether they receive drug or placebo, we can calculate the probability of observing a difference in healing rates between drug and placebo as large as or larger than 60/100 compared with 30/100. The sum is more complicated than in the coin tossing example, but it turns out that the probability of such an extreme difference is again small, $3 \cdot 7 \times 10^{-5}$ in fact. Put another way, if in ulcer patients overall there were a similar 45% healing rate whether they received drug or placebo, and we repeatedly carried out trials of similar design to our original study in samples of 200 patients, fewer than one in 10 000 of such trials would find a difference between drug and placebo as large as 60% compared with 30%.

Given that such an extreme outcome is so unlikely under our original assumption of no difference between drug and placebo, we might decide to reject the assumption and conclude instead that there is in fact a difference.

The approach that has been illustrated in the above two examples is the basis of statistical hypothesis testing. We start by making a *null hypothesis* about the population of interest (for example, that healing rates are no different in patients given drug or placebo). Often this hypothesis is the negation of the end point in which we are really interested (that drug treatment is better than placebo)—hence the "null" in the nomenclature. Next we make observations in a sample selected from the population. Usually the outcome in this sample will deviate somewhat from the null hypothesis. We then calculate the probability of obtaining a deviation from the null hypothesis as large as or larger than that which we have observed, simply through the chance variation that can be expected from one sample to another. This probability is commonly termed a *P value* or *level of statistical significance*. Thus a P value is defined as:

> The probability of obtaining an outcome as or more extreme than that observed in the study if the null hypothesis were true.

If a P value is low we may decide to reject the null hypothesis as incorrect.

Statistical significance

How low should a P value be before we reject the null hypothesis? There is no simple answer to this question. All we can say is that other things being equal, the lower the P value, the less credible the null hypothesis.

Traditionally, P values less than 0·05 have often been assigned special status and deemed *statistically significant*. However, there is nothing intrinsically unique about the level of 0·05, and the difference between P values of 0.049 and 0·051 is no more important than that between values of 0·047 and 0·049. The term 'statistically significant' is a literary convenience when describing results, but the fact that a finding is statistically significant does not mean that it cannot legitimately be attributed to chance. Indeed, if a large number of independent statistical tests are carried out (as is often the case in epidemiological studies), one in 20 can be expected to show statistical significance at a 5% level even if all of the null hypotheses are true. Nor does failure to achieve statistical significance preclude us from concluding that a null hypothesis is unlikely to be correct. The final conclusions from an analysis depend on other factors as well as the level of statistical significance attained—in particular, the design and size of the study and the weight of evidence from other investigations (see chapter 9).

One often sees P values quoted in relation to a reference—P<0·05, P<0·01, or P<0·001—but it is better if possible to give the exact P value—for example, P = 0·023 as this conveys more information (just as it is more informative to say that a car costs £11 500 than to quote the price as "under £12 000").

Statistical tests

In the example of the coin tossing experiment in which all ten tosses came out the same, calculation of the P value was fairly straightforward. Usually, however, the mathematics is more complex. For example, to compute the probability of obtaining at least seven tosses the same in a sequence of ten tosses requires application of more advanced techniques than can be covered in this book. For the same reason, in the comparison of ulcer healing rates between drug and placebo, the P value was quoted without an indication of how it was derived. Calculation of this P value from first principles would be extremely complicated.

Fortunately, the derivation of P values can usually be made easier by application of an appropriate *statistical test*. A statistical test can be viewed as a shorthand method of obtaining a P value. It entails calculation of a special summary statistic from the sample data according to a set formula or recipe (box 5.A), and then looking up this value of the statistic in a table which gives the corresponding P value. Nowadays, calculation of the statistic and its checking against tabulated values are normally carried out by computer.

There are many different statistical tests, each with its own special formula for calculating the relevant statistic and its own table for looking up P values (box 5.B). The choice of the correct test depends on the nature of the data, the study design, and the hypothesis under investigation. For example, different tests are applied to nominal, ordinal, and quantitative data.

Parametric and non-parametric tests

A broad distinction is made between parametric and non-parametric tests. A parametric test makes assumptions about the distribution of data in the population from which the study sample is drawn. For example, in a study comparing the birth weights of

67

Box 5.A   An example of the use of a statistical test

Suppose that a survey is carried out to find out whether attempted suicide is associated with unemployment, and that in a comparison of 100 cases of attempted suicide and 160 controls, the levels of unemployment are as in the contingency table:

	Cases	Controls	Total
Unemployed	36	16	52
Employed	64	144	208
Total	100	160	260

The proportion of cases unemployed (36/100 = 36%) is higher than that of controls (16/160 = 10%), but could this difference have occurred by chance?

The null hypothesis here is that there is no underlying difference in the unemployment rates of cases and controls in the population from which our sample of 260 subjects came. We assume that in the source population the observed overall unemployment rate (52/260 = 20%) applies equally to both cases and controls

The probability of observing such a large difference between cases and controls (36/100 v 16/160) if this null hypothesis were true can be calculated quickly by use of a statistical test, and in this particular case the appropriate test is the chi square test. The relevant statistic is calculated from the sample data according to a set formula:

$$\frac{N(\mid ad - bc \mid - N/2)^2}{(a+b)(c+d)(a+c)(b+d)}$$

where a is the number of unemployed cases, b of unemployed controls, c of employed cases and d of employed controls, N = a + b + c + d; and $\mid ad - bc \mid$ means ad − bc if ad is larger than bc and bc − ad if bc is larger than ad.

Thus, we here obtain a value for the statistic of

$$\frac{260((36 \times 144 - 16 \times 64) - 260/2)^2}{(36+16)(64+144)(36+100)(16+144)}$$

Continued

Box 5.A—*continued*

$$= \frac{260(5184 - 1024 - 130)^2}{52 \times 208 \times 100 \times 160}$$

$$= \frac{260 \times 4030^2}{52 \times 208 \times 100 \times 160}$$

$$= 24 \cdot 4$$

When we look this up in the relevant reference table we find that it corresponds to a P value of 8×10^{-7}

There are many statistical tests, each with its own special formula for deriving the relevant statistic and its own look-up table. Choosing the right statistical test for a particular problem requires experience, and doctors who are in doubt will do best to consult a statistician

Box 5.B   Some examples of statistical tests

Chi square (χ^2) test
McNemar's test
t test
Paired t test
Chi square test for trend
Variance ratio test (F test)
Mann–Whitney U test

babies whose mothers did or did not receive nutritional supplements during pregnancy, a parametric test might assume that the underlying distribution of birth weights was normal (Gaussian). Non-parametric tests make no assumptions of this kind. The advantage of parametric tests is that they allow stronger conclusions, provided that the assumptions which they make can be accepted.

Following the recipe for a test is not too difficult, but choosing the correct test for a particular set of data and study question requires skill and experience and is not a job for the amateur. Unless they can be confident in their own ability, doctors will do best to consult a medical statistician about which test to use. For those who are concerned only with interpreting other people's published analyses, it is more important to identify the null hypothesis under investigation and the P value obtained than to worry about the statistical test that was used to derive the P value. Concerns about the latter can be left to statistical referees who review papers before publication and to the minority of readers who are more knowledgeable in statistics.

One tailed and two tailed tests

Reports of statistical analyses in medical journals sometimes refer to tests of statistical significance as one tailed or two tailed. This distinction relates to the possibility that deviation from a null hypothesis can occur in two directions. For example, when we compare a drug with placebo in a clinical trial, our null hypothesis is that there is no underlying difference in outcome. Deviation from this hypothesis can occur because patients receiving the drug fare better than those receiving placebo, or vice versa. A one tailed or *one sided* test calculates the probability of deviation from the null hypothesis in a specified direction. Thus, with the assumption of no underlying difference between drug and placebo, we might derive the probability of observing a benefit from the drug relative to placebo as large as that found in our study. In contrast, a two tailed or *two sided* test calculates the probability of deviation from the null hypothesis in either direction—for example, the probability of a difference in outcome (beneficial or adverse) between drug and placebo as large as that observed.

Two tailed tests are more conservative than one tailed tests (for a given set of data they give higher P values) and are used more often. If a test in a published report is not specified as one tailed or two tailed, it is usually safe to assume that it is two tailed. The choice of which to use is a matter of personal taste, but the difference in their meaning must be borne in mind when results are interpreted.

70

Questions

5.1 What is the null hypothesis in a study:

(a) To find out whether use of a new surgical technique reduces rates of wound infection.

(b) To find out whether patients from fundholding general practices wait shorter times for outpatient appointments.

(c) To find out whether adenoidectomy reduces absence from school in children with middle ear disease.

5.2 What is meant by the P values in the following statements?

(a) In a trial of a new analgesic regimen used in terminal illness, patients reported more satisfactory pain relief than when receiving conventional treatment ($P = 0.02$).

(b) In a comparison of the workloads of two accident and emergency departments there was no significant difference in the numbers of hip fractures treated over a 12 month period ($P > 0.05$).

(c) Advice to mothers in a community not to leave babies face down in their cots was associated with a significant reduction ($P < 0.05$) in rates of sudden infant death over two years as compared with the two previous years.

6 Estimation with confidence intervals

In the example of the coin tossing experiment that was described in chapter 5, we were in effect looking at samples from the hypothetical population of all sequences of tosses that could be made with the coin under study. We considered two samples—one of three tosses, and the other of 10 tosses. The findings in both samples were the same insofar as all tosses were the same, but the P values were quite different—0·25 for the sample of three tosses as compared with approximately 0·002 for the sample of 10 tosses.

This illustrates an important feature of statistical significance. The statistical significance of a finding depends not only on the extent of its deviation from the null hypothesis (100% heads instead of 50% heads) but also on the size of the sample in which that deviation is observed. Consider two clinical trials comparing treatments for leukaemia, one involving 20 patients and the other 2000 patients. One measure of efficacy might be the proportion of patients going into remission (meaning that the peripheral blood count is normal and fewer than 5% of the nucleated cells in the bone marrow are blasts) after treatment. Table 6.1 shows the P values for two possible outcomes of such trials under the null hypothesis of no difference between the treatments. In the case of the first study, the observed benefit from treatment A is large (50% v 25% remission), but because this is observed in only a small sample of patients the P value is unremarkable. In contrast, the observed benefit from treatment A in the second study is much smaller (25% v 20%), but because of the larger sample size this is more significant statistically (P = 0·009).

In practice, when deciding which of two treatments for leukaemia to use, we need to know not only which is the better therapy but also by how much it is better. If the added benefit from a drug is minimal and its cost extortionate, then it is unlikely to be a

Table 6.1   Levels of statistical significance in two clinical trials of treatment for leukaemia

	Treatment A		Treatment B		Statistical significance of difference between A and B
	No of patients	No going into remission	No of patients	No going into remission	
Trial I	20	10	20	5	0·2
Trial II	1000	250	1000	200	0·009

treatment of choice. In the same way, if we had to decide how much resource to commit to a public health campaign promoting the use of sun creams to protect against skin cancer, we would need information on the extent to which sun exposure affects the risk of skin cancer, and not simply on whether or not there is a hazard. In general, decisions in medical practice depend not on whether an effect is present, but on how big the effect is.

It follows that hypothesis testing is not the most appropriate statistical technique for informing medical decisions. A finding that is highly significant statistically may be clinically irrelevant (because the effect is small). On the other hand, clinically important outcomes may fail to achieve statistical significance if they are observed only in small samples.

Because of this, the trend in recent years has been to an alternative approach to statistical inference using *estimation* with *confidence intervals*. From a study sample we can make an estimate of the outcome measure or effect in which we are interested (the difference in cure rates between two treatments, for example), but we are left with the problem that even if our sample has been properly selected, it may be atypical simply by chance. A confidence interval is a measure of how much trust we can place in an estimate derived from a sample, taking into account the scope for chance variation from one sample to another.

What are confidence intervals?

As with hypothesis testing, the concept of a confidence interval should be viewed in the context of a sample derived from a larger population about which conclusions are to be drawn. Specifically, there are numerical attributes or parameters of the population which we would like to estimate. Examples of such *population parameters* might be 'the percentage five-year survival of patients with newly diagnosed oesophageal cancer', 'the prevalence of Down's syndrome in babies born to mothers over 35 years of age', 'the risk of colonic cancer in patients who have had ulcerative colitis for more than 10 years', or 'the reduction in general practice consultation rates following introduction of a new policy for managing patients with asthma in the community'. Corresponding to each such population parameter is a *sample statistic*—for example, the percentage five-year survival in a sample of patients with newly diagnosed oesophageal cancer, the prevalence of Down's syndrome in a sample of babies born to mothers over 35 years of age, etc.

A sample statistic constitutes a *point estimate* of the corresponding population parameter. However, even if the sample has been chosen in an appropriate way, this estimate will not be completely reliable. If the same study were repeated with a different sample from the same population, the point estimate obtained would probably be different, just because of the chance variation between samples. In essence, a confidence interval gives a range around a point estimate within which the corresponding population parameter is likely to lie (assuming that the study has been well designed and conducted).

Most often, 95% confidence intervals are quoted. A 95% confidence interval for an estimate is derived from the sample data according to set mathematical rules. Its meaning can be better understood if we consider the theoretical situation in which a study is repeated a large number of times, using different samples selected from the same population. Each sample will produce its own point estimate and surrounding confidence interval, and some of these confidence intervals will include the population parameter while others do not (see box 6.A(a)). The mathematical recipe for deriving the 95% confidence intervals is set so that, in the long run, 95% of samples will have confidence intervals that include the population parameter.

Sometimes 90% confidence intervals are given instead. The rules for calculating 90% confidence intervals are set in such a way that in a large series of samples, each with its own confidence interval, 90% of confidence intervals will include the corresponding population parameter. It follows that for a given sample, the 90% confidence interval will be narrower than the 95% confidence interval (box 6.A (b))

Box 6.A Confidence intervals

(a) If a study were repeated a large number of times using different samples selected from the same population, each sample would produce its own 95% confidence interval

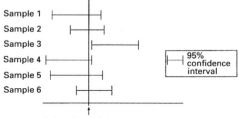

Value of population parameter

In the above example the 95% CI for sample 3 does not include the population parameter that is being estimated. The formula for calculating 95% confidence intervals is set in such a way that in the long run 95% of such confidence intervals will include the population parameter (assuming that the study is well designed and executed)

(b) 90% confidence intervals are narrower than the corresponding 95% confidence intervals and are derived according to a formula such that on average 90% of such intervals will include the population parameter

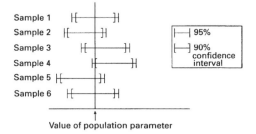

Value of population parameter

Here the 90% confidence interval for sample 4 excludes the population parameter, but the corresponding 95% confidence interval does not

The methods of calculating confidence intervals depend on the type of data that is being analysed (nominal, ordinal, or quantitative), the design of the study, and the parameter that is being estimated. Computer programs are available for calculating confidence intervals, but choosing the right method requires skill and experience; if in doubt, doctors do best to consult a medical statistician.

The relation of confidence intervals to P values

A null hypothesis can be viewed as postulating a null value for a population parameter. For example, the null hypothesis that there is no difference in cure rates between two drugs is equivalent to a proposition that the parameter representing the difference in cure rates between the two drugs has a value of zero. If we obtain a result that is statistically significant with a P value of less than 0·05, this is equivalent (at least to a close approximation) to a statement that the 95% confidence interval for the relevant population parameter does not include the postulated null value.

Suppose, for example, that an epidemiological study is carried out to investigate the association of smoking with cervical cancer. The null hypothesis in this case is that no association exists—that the population parameter defined as the ratio of cervical cancer rates in smokers and non-smokers has a value of one. A statement that an association was found between smoking and cervical cancer with a P value of less than 0·05 is equivalent to saying that the 95% confidence interval for the estimated ratio of cervical cancer rates in smokers and non-smokers did not include one.

Because of this equivalence, P values tell us little extra when confidence intervals are known.

Standard error

Sometimes estimates of population parameters are quoted with their standard errors rather than confidence intervals. A standard error is a statistic calculated from measurements in a sample, often as an intermediate step in the derivation of a confidence interval or P value. In particular, where a sample mean is used to estimate a population mean, the upper and lower 95% confidence limits (the upper and lower bounds of the 95% confidence interval) are given approximately by the sample mean plus or minus twice its standard error (the exact calculation depends on the size of the sample).

Thus, in a sample of men aged 16–64 the mean difference in daily vitamin C intake between non-smokers and heavy smokers was 19·2 mg with a standard error of 7·8 mg. It follows that the 95% confidence interval for the estimated mean difference in vitamin C intakes by smoking habit in the population from which these men came is approximately $19·2 - (2 \times 7·8)$ to $19·2 + (2 \times 7·8)$ —that is, 3·6 to 34·8 mg.

In general, confidence intervals can be interpreted more directly than standard errors and are a preferable method of presenting results.

Sample size and confidence intervals

Other things being equal, the larger the size of a sample, the narrower the confidence interval that will be obtained. This reflects the fact that bigger samples provide more information and therefore allow more confident conclusions with a smaller range of uncertainty. This theme will be developed further in the next chapter.

Questions

6.1 In follow up of men who participated in nuclear weapons tests, leukaemia mortality was 1·75 times that in a control group (95% confidence interval 1·01 to 3·06).

(a) What is meant by this 95% confidence interval?

(b) Would the excess mortality in the study group as compared with controls be statistically significant (P<0·05)?

6.2 In an analysis of controlled trials of nicotine replacement as an aid to smoking cessation, nicotine chewing gum had an efficacy (defined as the difference in percentages of treated and control subjects who had stopped smoking at one year) of 6% (95% confidence interval 4% to 8%).

(a) What does this confidence interval mean?

(b) How could a narrower 95% confidence interval be obtained?

7 Statistical power and selection of samples

With a given study design, larger samples provide more information. This was illustrated in the coin-tossing experiment described in chapter 5. With a sample of only three tosses it was not possible to draw any worthwhile conclusions about the fairness of the coin, whereas the result of 10 tosses brought the fairness of the coin into serious doubt. Small samples are more often unrepresentative by chance, and therefore do not allow such confident conclusions as large samples.

This is reflected by wider confidence intervals when samples are small. Box 7.A shows confidence intervals in three drug trials. In

---

Box 7.A Effect of sample size on confidence intervals

Consider three trials comparing a drug with placebo and using mortality as an outcome measure. The table below shows the 95% confidence intervals that would be associated with a reduction in mortality of 5% according to the size of sample in which it was observed

	Placebo		Drug		Reduction in mortality with drug as compared with placebo	
	No of patients	No of deaths	No of patients	No of deaths	Point estimate	95% confidence interval
Trial I	40	10	40	8	5%	−13% to +23%
Trial II	400	100	400	80	5%	−1% to +11%
Trial III	1600	400	1600	320	5%	+2% to +8%

The larger the sample size, the narrower the confidence interval

---

each trial there is an estimated reduction in mortality of 5% with the drug as compared with placebo, but the confidence intervals around this estimate vary enormously according to the size of the study. With only 40 patients in each treatment group, there is major uncertainty about the apparent benefit from the drug. Indeed, the findings would be quite compatible with its having a detrimental effect as compared with placebo. On the other hand, the benefit could easily be as much as a 23% reduction in mortality. In contrast, the largest study provides a much more precise estimate of benefit, indicating that it probably lies in the range 2% to 8%. We say that this study has more *power*.

In essence, the power of a study is its ability to minimise the uncertainties that arise because of chance variation between samples. Two methods are commonly used to quantify power. Once a study has been completed, confidence intervals provide the most convenient and easily interpreted measure of power. They tell us with how big and how small values for the parameter of interest the findings could easily be compatible. However, confidence intervals do not lend themselves so readily to the advance quantification of power when studies are being planned. In this case the usual approach is to base power calculations on the hypothesis testing approach to statistical inference.

Type 1 and type 2 error

When hypothesis testing is carried out, two sorts of error can occur. First, the null hypothesis may be rejected when in fact it is true. This is called *type 1* or *alpha* error. Alternatively, the null hypothesis may escape rejection when in reality it is incorrect. This is termed *type 2* or *beta* error.

There is an inverse relation between the probabilities of type 1 and type 2 error. Thus, if stringent criteria are set for rejecting the null hypothesis (a P value of less than $0 \cdot 001$, say), the chance of type 1 error will (by definition) be lower than with a less demanding threshold (for example, a P value of less than $0 \cdot 05$). On the other hand, the chance of type 2 error will be higher. This is illustrated in box 7.B, which shows how the probability of type 2 error might vary across a range of thresholds for rejecting the null hypothesis in a clinical trial.

Box 7.B   Probability of type 2 error in relation to thresholds for rejecting the null hypothesis in a clinical trial

The figure illustrates the relation between the probability of type 2 error and the level of statistical significance at which the null hypothesis will be rejected for three clinical trials comparing a drug with placebo. In each case it is assumed that equal numbers of patients are randomised to drug and placebo, and that the drug halves mortality from 20% to 10%. However, the trials differ in the total number (N) of patients studied

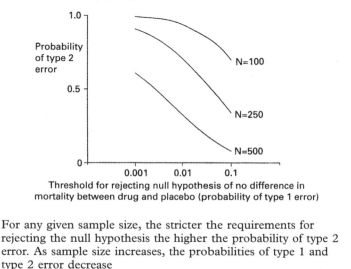

For any given sample size, the stricter the requirements for rejecting the null hypothesis the higher the probability of type 2 error. As sample size increases, the probabilities of type 1 and type 2 error decrease

---

Given the threshold at which the null hypothesis will be rejected, studies with greater power have a lower probability of type 2 error. Thus, the quantity defined as one minus the probability of type 2 error can be taken as a measure of power.* We might say that a study will have 80% power to detect an effect of a given size at a 5% level of statistical significance, meaning that if we set the

---

* Technically, the measure is termed the "statistical power" of the study. I have used the term "power" in a more general sense to describe the quality of which "statistical power" is one measure.

threshold for rejecting the null hypothesis at a P value of 5% then the probability of type 2 error will be $(100 - 80)\% = 20\%$. This index of power will depend on:

- sample size—bigger studies have greater statistical power;
- the extent to which the null hypothesis is incorrect—if the true state of affairs is very different from the null hypothesis then the study is more likely to produce a low P value and the null hypothesis is less likely to be accepted in error;
- certain features of the study population, according to the design of the study.

For example, in a case-control study examining the relation of acute upper gastrointestinal bleeding to recent aspirin intake, the null hypothesis would postulate the same prevalence of aspirin use in cases and in controls without bleeding. The statistical power of the study to detect an association between aspirin and bleeding, measured as one minus the probability of type 2 error, would depend on the threshold for rejecting the null hypothesis, the numbers of cases and controls, the strength of the true association (measured as an odds ratio†) and the prevalence of aspirin use in controls. Table 7.1 gives some examples of how these different variables would influence the power. If an investigator planning such a study could specify the threshold that would be used to reject the null hypothesis, the level of the odds ratio that it was important to detect, and the likely prevalence of aspirin use in controls, then levels of power could be calculated for different numbers of cases and controls, and an appropriate sample size could be chosen.

In a study comparing mean systolic blood pressures in people on a low salt diet and on a normal diet, the null hypothesis would be that there is no difference in mean systolic pressures. Here the power would depend on the threshold for rejecting the null hypothesis, the number of subjects, the true difference in blood pressure associated with a low salt diet, and the variability of blood pressures between different people when on a normal diet

---

† The ratio of the odds of upper gastrointestinal bleeding in someone who has recently taken aspirin to those in someone who has not. This is a measure of the extent to which aspirin is associated with an increased risk of bleeding. For example, an odds ratio of two would imply that gastrointestinal bleeding was approximately twice as common in recent users of aspirin as in non-users.

Table 7.1 Factors influencing the power of a case-control study to detect an association between recent aspirin intake and acute upper gastrointestinal bleeding

True odds ratio	Threshold for rejecting null hypothesis	Prevalence of recent aspirin intake in controls	No of cases	No of controls	Power (%)
2·0	P = 0·01	10%	50	50	4
2·0	P = 0·01	10%	100	100	12
2·0	P = 0·01	10%	100	200	16
2·0	P = 0·05	10%	50	50	14
2·0	P = 0·05	10%	100	100	30
2·0	P = 0·05	10%	100	200	38
2·0	P = 0·05	20%	50	50	76
2·0	P = 0·05	20%	100	100	98
2·0	P = 0·05	20%	100	200	100
4·0	P = 0·01	10%	50	50	39
4·0	P = 0·01	10%	100	100	83
4·0	P = 0·01	10%	100	200	94
4·0	P = 0·05	10%	50	50	68
4·0	P = 0·05	10%	100	100	95
4·0	P = 0·05	10%	100	200	99
4·0	P = 0·05	20%	50	50	99
4·0	P = 0·05	20%	100	100	100
4·0	P = 0·05	20%	100	200	100

(measured as their standard deviation). Table 7.2 shows how these factors interrelate.

When planning studies it is important to ensure that they will have adequate power, or time and effort will be wasted in a fruitless exercise. Because the methods of calculating power vary according to the study design, doctors will normally do best to seek help from a medical statistician. In doing so, however, they should be prepared to define a null hypothesis and the extent of deviation from this that they would hope to detect. They must also be ready to answer questions about the likely distribution of key variables in their study population. The statistician will explain which variable or variables are relevant, according to the study design.

Selecting samples

Once an adequate sample size has been calculated, the method by which the sample is chosen may be straightforward. For example, in a hospital-based clinical trial, eligible patients would normally be recruited consecutively until the required number had been

Table 7.2 Factors influencing the power of a study to detect a difference in systolic blood pressure between people on a low salt diet and an equal number of people on a normal diet

True mean reduction in systolic pressure (mm Hg)	Threshold for rejecting null hypothesis	Standard deviation of systolic pressures in people on a normal diet (mm Hg)	Total no of subjects	Power (%)
2	P = 0·01	15	100	3
2	P = 0·01	15	200	5
2	P = 0·01	15	400	11
2	P = 0·01	10	100	6
2	P = 0·01	10	200	12
2	P = 0·01	10	400	28
2	P = 0·05	15	100	10
2	P = 0·05	15	200	15
2	P = 0·05	15	400	27
2	P = 0·05	10	100	17
2	P = 0·05	10	200	29
2	P = 0·05	10	400	52
4	P = 0·05	15	100	27
4	P = 0·05	15	200	47
4	P = 0·05	15	400	76
4	P = 0·05	10	100	52
4	P = 0·05	10	200	81
4	P = 0·05	10	400	98

obtained; and in a case-control study of patients with asthma from a general practice it might be necessary to include all available cases in order to achieve satisfactory numbers. Sometimes, however, there is a pool of potential subjects from which only a proportion is needed. For example, in a survey to compare the prevalence of back pain in adults from eight areas of Britain, power calculations indicated that it would be necessary to study only one in 20 local residents in order to have a good chance of detecting any important differences in the occurrence of back disorders.

In this case, the way in which the study sample is chosen from the *study population* of eligible subjects is critical to the validity of subsequent statistical inference. Various methods of sampling can be used, some better than others.

Quota sampling

In market research the technique of quota sampling is often used. The study population is divided into bands or strata according to criteria such as age, sex, and socioeconomic group, and target quotas are set for each stratum with the aim of obtaining a representative mix of people in the study sample. For example, 30 men and 30 women might be required in each of the age bands 20–39, 40–59, and 60 +. The investigator then approaches people, perhaps in the street or by telephoning addresses sequentially, until the quotas are filled.

The weakness of this method is that certain sectors of the study population may be systematically excluded from the sample (for example, people too busy to answer questions on the street or those who do not have a telephone), leading to serious bias. Quota sampling is therefore rarely used in medical research.

Systematic sampling

More acceptable is to take a systematic sample—for example, every tenth person from a list of all members of the study population. But this is still not ideal. Bias may arise because of the way in which subjects are ordered in the listing of the study population. Thus, in an age-sex register of a general practice any twins of the same sex will appear consecutively, and a systematic sample would never pick up both members of a pair. Depending on the purpose of the study, this could lead to error.

Also, the investigator may be tempted to manipulate the order of the population listing so that some subjects are deliberately included in or excluded from the sample, and this could render the sample unrepresentative.

Simple random sampling

These weaknesses are overcome by use of random sampling methods. By *random sampling* we mean that each member of the study population has a defined, non-zero probability of being included in the study sample. In simple random sampling all subjects have an equal probability of inclusion. For example, a sample might be chosen so that each subject had a random, one in 15 chance of selection.

The starting point for random sampling is an ordered listing of the study population. This listing is known as the *sampling frame*. If the study population comprised the patients registered with a general practice, an age-sex register would provide a suitable sampling frame. In a study of women who had undergone hysterectomy at a hospital during a specified period, the sampling frame could be based on a list of all such operations, ordered according to the date and time at which they were carried out. The method by which the sampling frame is ordered is entirely a matter of convenience. Any ordering will do, but it must be defined at the outset.

Next, the sample is selected from the listing by use of *random numbers*. Random numbers are a sequence of digits generated by computer according to a special mathematical formula. Technically speaking, numbers derived in this way are not truly random, but to all intents and purposes they behave as if they were random. In the long run, each digit from zero to nine appears with equal frequency, and no sequence of two, three, or four digits occurs more frequently than any other of the same length. Box 7.C shows an extract from a table of random numbers. Such tables can be found published in books of statistical tables and in many statistical textbooks.

Suppose that we wish to select a sample of 20 subjects from a population of 90. This could be done using a table such as that in box 7.C. First, we decide how the table is to be read—from left to right in rows working down the page is a natural method, given that this is how we normally read text. Next, a starting point in the table is chosen by shutting the eyes and placing the point of a pencil on the page. Let us assume that the starting point is the number 07 underlined in box 7.C.

Our sampling frame allows us to allocate each member of the study population a two digit number from 01 to 90. Therefore, beginning at our chosen starting point, we read off a series of two digit numbers from the table. The first number is 07, so this subject enters the sample, followed by subjects 61, 58, and 85. The next number, 98, lies outside the range 01 to 90, so we simply ignore it and go on to the next. Similarly, if a subject already selected came up a second time, we would just go on to the next number. We continue in this way until we have the 20 subjects that we need.

This may at first seem an unnecessarily laborious approach to sample selection. Why not just pick 20 subjects from the 90 in a seemingly haphazard manner? Unfortunately, such haphazard methods tend on average to be far from random, and only proper random sampling can be guaranteed free from systematic error.

Box 7.C Extract from a table of random numbers

44	32	21	24	15	60	05	31	38	54	96	84
21	47	96	61	08	19	58	47	18	75	42	24
15	58	41	69	43	25	72	53	45	27	66	58
41	07	61	58	85	98	31	78	34	67	50	06
10	29	76	10	70	45	33	95	86	72	49	84
66	69	12	96	42	01	38	53	30	51	57	04
66	24	90	33	53	15	41	19	15	11	77	79
62	50	42	40	99	02	95	34	37	08	13	77
86	14	77	44	14	02	79	41	04	12	00	28

For ease of reading, the digits are grouped in pairs, but they can be read in sequences of any required length (single digits, pairs, triplets etc). For a description of how such a table could be used to select a random sample, see text.

These days the process of selecting random samples has been made easier because most personal computers are fitted with software that will generate random numbers. Thus, a fairly simple program can be written to list 20 numbers at random between 01 and 90 without any need to look up tables of random numbers. Doctors needing to select large random samples (of size greater than 100, say) may find it worthwhile to seek help from a statistician or computer programmer.

Stratified random sampling

Sometimes the investigator wishes to fix the distribution of certain characteristics in the study sample—for example, the numbers of men and women. This is achieved by stratified random sampling. The study population is partitioned into strata according to the characteristics concerned, and simple random sampling is carried out within each stratum to obtain the required numbers. So, the male members of the study population might be randomly sampled to obtain 40 men, and the female members to obtain 40 women.

With stratified random sampling, members of the study population do not necessarily all have the same probability of inclusion in the study sample. Some strata may be relatively over-represented by design. Thus, to permit subsidiary analyses of

---

Box 7.D   Stratified random sampling

Suppose that we wish to select a sample of 200 people from a population of 1000 with an age distribution as shown below:

Age group	Population
20–39	500
40–59	400
60+	100
All ages	1000

If we select a simple random sample with a sampling fraction of one in five then we can expect only 20 members of our sample to be aged 60+ years. This will limit statistical power to draw any conclusions about this age band. An alternative would be to select a stratified random sample as shown below:

Age group	Population	Sampling fraction	Sample
20–39	500	14 per 100	70
40–59	400	17·5 per 100	70
60+	100	60 per 100	60

Relative oversampling from the oldest age group might ensure an adequate sample size in each age band.

---

adequate statistical power in different age groups, a sample could be stratified by age with deliberately enhanced representation of the elderly, who otherwise might be too few in number (box 7.D).

Multistage sampling

Sometimes, especially in epidemiological studies, it is more convenient or economical to carry out random sampling in two or more stages. For example, suppose that the study population comprises residents of a large city. To compile a suitable sampling frame for the full study population could be difficult. An alternative might be first to select a random sample of general practices from all the practices in the city, and then to select random samples of patients from the lists of the chosen practices. This is called *multistage* or *cluster sampling*. Provided the number of practices selected was not too few, and a similar proportion of patients was sampled from each list, such a sample should be reasonably representative.

Randomisation in clinical trials

A special case of sampling is the allocation of patients to different treatments in clinical trials. From the population of all patients included in the study, samples must be selected for each treatment. To avoid bias, this again is best achieved by random selection. In prospective studies the sampling frame is usually established according to the order in which patients are recruited to the study, and random numbers are then used to assign the patients to different treatment groups.

Suppose, for example, that there are two treatments, A and B, under comparison, and we would like roughly equal numbers of patients to receive each. A sequence of random numbers could be generated by computer or abstracted from a table of random numbers. If the first number were odd, the first patient would receive treatment A, and if it were even, treatment B would be given. The treatment for the second patient would be determined in a similar way from the second number in the series (odd for treatment A and even for treatment B) and so on.

Modifications of this technique can be applied to distribute patients between any number of treatments. It is important, however, that the investigator does not know which treatment will be allocated by the randomisation until after the patient has been assigned a place in the sampling frame. Otherwise, there is a danger that entry to the study will be manipulated deliberately or subconsciously so that certain patients are treated according to the investigator's wishes rather than at random. For example, in a trial of self-administered physiotherapy after stroke, the investigator might prefer less motivated patients to receive conventional treatment, believing that they would not comply adequately with the self-administered regimen. Knowing that the next person to enter the trial would receive self-administered therapy, he might be disinclined to recruit a poorly motivated patient, preferring to treat such a patient conventionally outside the trial. However, he would happily recruit the same patient if he knew that the next assigned treatment in the trial would be conventional therapy. In the long run, the outcome of such a policy would be to allocate a higher proportion of well motivated patients to the self-administered therapy than to conventional treatment, and this could produce a misleading outcome. If the outcome of randomisation is revealed only after a subject has entered the study, this problem is avoided.

Questions

7.1 What sampling frames might be used to select a sample of 11 year old children living in the city of Winchester?

7.2 The figure below shows how the statistical power (given as a percentage of the maximum achievable given the number of cases) of a case-control study relates to the ratio of controls to cases when other variables (including the number of cases) are fixed.

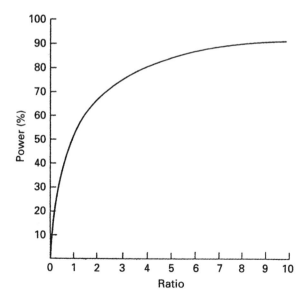

What implications does this have for sampling strategies in case-control studies?

7.3 In writing a grant proposal for a trial to evaluate behaviour therapy in the treatment of sleep disorders, how might you specify the power of the study?

7.4 In reporting the results of a trial to evaluate behaviour therapy in the treatment of sleep disorders, how might you specify the power of the study?

7.5 In a report of a comparison of lung cancer rates between coal miners and dockers it was stated that there were no statistically significant differences in the smoking habits of the two occupational groups. Why is this use of statistical significance unsatisfactory?

8 Statistical modelling

Statistical analyses reported in medical journals often make use of statistical models. A statistical model starts with specified assumptions about the interrelation of different variables in the study population and estimates population parameters, or derives P values from sample data on the basis of these assumptions. For example, one modelling technique that is commonly applied is that of multiple linear regression.

Multiple linear regression

Table 8.1 shows an extract of data on lung function from a cross sectional survey of 276 men and women aged 65 years and older. For each subject there is a measurement of forced expiratory ratio (FEV_1/FVC), and also a record of age, sex, and smoking habits. We might ask how important are age, sex, and smoking habits as predictors of forced expiratory ratio.

Table 8.1 Extract of data on lung function from a cross sectional survey of 276 men and women aged 65 years and older

Subject No	Age (years)	Sex	Smoking habit	Forced expiratory ratio (FEV_1/FVC (%))
1	71	M	Smoker	47
2	88	M	Smoker	56
3	83	F	Never smoked	74
4	71	M	Smoker	70
5	67	F	Smoker	71
6	81	F	Never smoked	76
7	68	F	Smoker	76
8	67	F	Smoker	41
9	75	F	Never smoked	75
10	83	F	Smoker	60
11	81	M	Smoker	68
12	73	M	Smoker	39

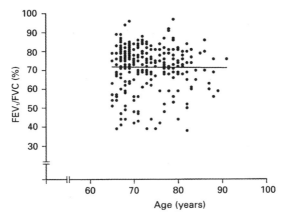

Figure 8.1 *Scatter plot of FEV₁/FVC against age*

This plot is based on the data which were illustrated in table 8.1. The regression line of FEV₁/FVC on age is marked, although the correlation is poor. The poor correlation is reflected in a relatively wide confidence interval for Parameter₁ in the multiple regression analysis (see text)

If we were looking only at age we could start by constructing a scatter plot as in figure 8.1, and we could derive an equation for the regression line of forced expiratory ratio on age. With the commonly adopted assumption that the ratio declines in a linear fashion with age (has a straight line relation to age), the slope of the regression line would give an estimate of the rate at which the ratio declines with age in the population from which the study sample was drawn.

Multiple linear regression extends this approach, allowing us to assess the importance of several variables simultaneously—in this case age, sex, and smoking habit. The simplest model would assume that forced expiratory ratio is predicted as the sum of four terms. The first is a baseline value. The second is a population parameter multiplied by the subject's age. This parameter represents the change in forced expiratory ratio associated with a one year increase in age. The third term is zero if the subject is a man, but takes the value of a second parameter if the subject is a woman. It indicates the difference in forced expiratory ratio between women and men. The last term is zero if the subject is a non-smoker and takes the value of a third parameter if he or she has smoked. It represents the difference in forced expiratory ratio

93

Box 8.A   Multiple linear regression for forced expiratory ratio (FEV_1/FVC (%))

	Point estimate	95% Confidence interval
Parameter$_1$ (effect of age)	−0·12	−0·35 to +0·10
Parameter$_2$ (effect of gender)	+4·12	+1·29 to +6·96
Parameter$_3$ (effect of smoking)	−5·44	−8·38 to −2·50

between smokers and non-smokers. In other words, we assume that the ratio is predicted as

baseline value
plus   Parameter$_1$ × (age in years)
plus   Parameter$_2$ × (0 if subject is male or 1 if female)
plus   Parameter$_3$ × (0 if subject is a non-smoker or 1 if a smoker)

The three population parameters can be estimated from the sample data with 95% confidence intervals. The results of the calculation are shown in box 8.A (we do not need to worry here about exactly how the calculations were carried out).

For example, from this analysis we would estimate that, given the sex and smoking habits of a subject, forced expiratory ratio falls by 0·12 percentage points for each year of age; and that with the age and sex of the subject given, the ratio is reduced by 5·44 percentage points if he or she has been a smoker. The corresponding confidence intervals indicate the range of values for these parameters with which the study findings would readily be compatible. Thus, in the absence of bias, the reduction in forced expiratory ratio associated with having smoked is likely to lie in the range 2·50 to 8·38 percentage points.

Put in this way, the results are not too difficult to understand, but they do depend on the assumptions of the model. For example, it is supposed that, given a person's smoking habits, forced expiratory ratio falls at the same constant rate with increasing age in both men and women. It is for the doctor to decide whether this makes sense biologically. From what is known about lung function, is it plausible that forced expiratory ratio would decline

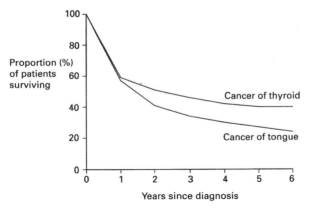

Figure 8.2 *Survival from diagnosis in male patients with cancer of the thyroid and cancer of the tongue*

at a roughly constant rate with increasing age, and that this rate would be similar in men and women? The statistician can test the validity of the assumptions to some extent using the study data, but the doctor must also evaluate them in the light of what is known from elsewhere.

Survival analyses

Another common application of statistical models is in the analysis of survival data. Many studies measure the 'survival' time from an initial event such as the diagnosis of a disease or start of a treatment until a specified outcome such as death, recovery, or discharge from hospital. One way of summarising the findings for a sample of patients is by means of a *survival curve*. For example, the survival curves in fig 8.2 show proportions of men with thyroid and tongue cancer who were still alive at different intervals after diagnosis.

Often the patients in a study of survival are not all followed for the same length of time. For example, in an investigation to assess the outcome of surgery for rectal cancer, patients would normally remain under surveillance from the time of their operation until they died or until the end of the study, whichever came sooner. In general, patients with operations early in the course of the study would be followed for longer than those who came under observation only shortly before the close of data collection. At first glance, it might seem that, for the purposes of statistical inference, patients who had been followed for only one year by the end of the study could not tell us anything useful about the chances of surviving 10 years from surgery. However, this is incorrect. Actuarial methods of *lifetable analysis* allow full use to be made of the data from all patients in the study.

The methods of lifetable analysis are too complex to describe in detail in a text of this length, but the general approach can be outlined. In the example above, the analysis might start by estimating the probability that a patient will survive one year from the date of operation. All patients would contribute to this calculation, with a small adjustment to take account of those who were not followed for a full year. Next, the findings for patients who were alive and being followed up one year after surgery would be used to estimate the probability of surviving a second year, assuming that death did not occur in the first 12 months. In a similar way, estimates would be obtained for the probabilities of surviving each successive year of follow up. Finally, the chances of surviving 10 years from surgery would be calculated by multiplying the estimated probabilities of surviving each year in turn:

(Probability of surviving from operation to year 1) × (probability of surviving from year 1 to year 2) × . . . × (probability of surviving from year 9 to year 10).

The probability of surviving a specified period from the date of operation is a population parameter for which the data from a study sample provide an estimate. By appropriate statistical techniques it is also possible to derive a 95% confidence interval for the estimate. In the example considered above, survival was measured until death, but the same methods could be applied to look at survival until other endpoints.

Sometimes survival is summarised by a single statistic such as a *12 month survival rate*—the proportion of patients surviving 12 months from entry to follow up without experiencing the endpoint of interest. However, a statistic of this sort conveys less information than a full survival curve. For example, in figure 8.2 thyroid and tongue cancer are both associated with a 12 month survival rate of just less than 60%. However, survival to six years is much lower for tongue cancer than for thyroid cancer.

In epidemiological studies and in the analysis of controlled trials we often wish to compare the survival curves of two or more groups of patients. For example, in a trial of a new immunosuppressant regimen for renal transplants we might compare the survival from transplantation to a first rejection episode with that of patients receiving conventional therapy. One statistical model that is commonly applied in this situation is a *proportional hazards analysis*. In its simplest form, this model assumes that at any given time after entry to follow up the probability of the outcome of interest (in this case rejection) in one group of patients (those receiving the new treatment) is a constant multiple of that in another group (those receiving conventional therapy). The ratio of probabilities is known as the *hazard ratio* and is a population parameter. It can be estimated from the findings in a study sample with an associated 95% confidence interval. In the study of immunosuppressants, a hazard ratio less than unity would imply that patients on the new treatment survived free of rejection for longer than those on conventional treatment.

Multiple regression and proportional hazards analysis are only two examples of the many models that may be employed in statistical inference. The same principles apply to the use of any model. When assessing the results, doctors should identify the assumptions underlying the model and assess their biological plausibility before drawing conclusions.

Questions

8.1 A statistician working with a doctor on a comparison of two treatment regimens for femoral neck fracture explains that she has used a proportional hazards model to compare survival in the two treatment groups. The model assumes that at any given time after starting treatment, the probability of death in the first treatment group is a constant multiple of the corresponding probability in the second treatment group. She has estimated this ratio and calculated a 95% confidence interval for it. What biological considerations might lead the doctor to question this model?

9 Interpretation of statistical analyses

Doctors who are not themselves carrying out research need an understanding of statistics mainly so that they can interpret other people's papers that are presented at meetings and in journals. Descriptive statistics are usually not too difficult to follow, but statistical inference presents more of a problem. Many of the analyses reported in medical journals use mathematical techniques that are beyond most clinicians, and there is a danger that results are either rejected as incomprehensible or accepted uncritically. A more constructive approach is to treat statistical analyses in a similar way to biochemical tests. It is not necessary to know all the technicalities of an assay for serum potassium in order to apply its results in clinical practice. However, the doctor does need to understand the implications of different potassium concentrations, and be able to interpret results in the light of other available clinical data—deciding, for example, whether a high concentration results from renal failure, an adverse effect of a drug, or simply a haemolysed specimen. In the same way, when assessing the findings of a clinical trial it is not essential to master all the mathematical nuances of survival analyses, but it is important to appreciate what is meant by an estimated 10% increase in five year survival and by the associated confidence interval. The doctor should be able to recognise shortcomings in the study method which might have led to error and should be able to interpret results in the light of data from other related studies.

The evaluation of studies that entail statistical inference is easier if a systematic approach is adopted. The first step is to identify the questions that are being asked and the population and circumstances in which the questions are being addressed. For example, in a study of prognosis in diabetic patients, is the focus on insulin dependent diabetes, non-insulin dependent diabetes, or both, and are there any restrictions in terms of age and sex? If hypothesis testing has been used, what are the null hypotheses under test? If estimation has been carried out, what are the population parameters of interest?

Assessment of bias

The next stage is to assess any biases that might be present. A *bias* is a deficiency in the design or execution of a study which leads a parameter to be systematically overestimated or systematically underestimated, or which tends to make P values falsely high or low. For example, in an epidemiological study of non-Hodgkin's lymphoma, cases were compared with controls who did not have the disease and subjects were asked if they had ever worked with organic solvents. The null hypothesis was of no association between non-Hodgkin's lymphoma and exposure to solvents, and the parameter to be estimated was the odds ratio of non-Hodgkin's lymphoma in people who have worked with solvents (effectively the ratio of their lymphoma risk to that of people with no exposure to solvents). If cases tended to recall past solvent use more completely than controls (perhaps because they were more interested in the study and better motivated), this would produce a bias. The odds ratio of non-Hodgkin's lymphoma from working with solvents would be exaggerated, and the null hypothesis of no association might be incorrectly rejected because of a spuriously low P value.

In searching for potential biases it is important to consider the selection of subjects or material for inclusion in the study. Is the study sample likely to be representative (as regards the study question) of the population to which the results will be applied?

Also, the reliability of measurements must be assessed. In the example of the lymphoma case-control study there was a possibility of bias because of errors in the ascertainment of solvent exposure. Quite often, studies suffer from missing data because measurements are not possible for all subjects in the study sample. This too may be a source of bias.

A potential for bias does not mean that a study should automatically be rejected as flawed. When investigations are carried out on human subjects, practical and ethical constraints often militate against an ideal study design, and a purist approach would lead to unnecessary loss of useful information. Rather, biases should be identified and their potential impact evaluated. In what direction are they likely to affect P values or estimates of parameters and how much?

For example, in a study of elderly men and women registered with three general practices the prevalence of respiratory symptoms was estimated by means of a postal questionnaire. Twenty eight per cent of those who replied to the questionnaire reported wheeze in the past year, but because only 83% of subjects responded, this prevalence estimate may have been biased. In particular, it is possible that symptom free patients were less inclined to participate, in which case an overestimate would have occurred. The reader must decide how much of an overestimate would be plausible, and interpret the result accordingly. (In the extreme case, none of the non-responders would have had wheeze, in which case the true prevalence in the study sample would have been 24%).

Assessment of chance error

The next step is to assess the potential for error because the study sample might be unrepresentative by chance. Confidence intervals and P values contribute importantly to this assessment, and their meanings have already been explained. The tighter the confidence interval, the more certain an estimate of a population parameter; and the lower the P value, the less credible a null hypothesis. Note, however, that confidence intervals and P values tell us only about chance effects; they do not allow for bias. An apparently precise estimate of a population parameter (one with a narrow confidence interval) may be wildly out if serious bias is present.

If the reader is not competent to assess the methods by which confidence intervals or P values have been derived then these must be accepted on trust. This is reasonable, especially when journals routinely employ statistical referees to check that calculations are appropriate.

Judgments about the likely contribution of chance to findings are helped by confidence intervals and P values, but these are not the only considerations. It is also important to set the results of a study in the context of what is known from other sources. If they diverge greatly from the findings of other investigations, we may conclude that they are unrepresentative even if the confidence interval is very tight or the P value very low. For example, if we carried out a study which showed a statistically significant (P<0·05) protective effect of smoking against lung cancer and there were no biases to explain this anomalous result, we might quite reasonably conclude that it had arisen by chance, despite its statistical significance. Put another way, given current knowledge, it would take an awful lot to convince us that smoking protects anyone from lung cancer.

How much weight is given to the results of other studies is subjective. So too is the assessment of bias. Even experts will disagree on the importance of a bias and on the strength of evidence from one investigation as compared with another. But then experts do not always agree on clinical matters either—the presence of a faint heart murmur or the optimal treatment for mild depression, for example. We have to live with the uncertainty. Where disagreements occur in the interpretation of studies, an understanding of statistical principles will help the doctor to identify the sources of discord and come to a conclusion.

Meta-analysis

Although assessment of the overall weight of evidence on a question will always be to some extent subjective, it may be possible to bring together the results from several similar studies in a formal meta-analysis. In a meta-analysis the data from two or more studies are pooled and analysed to produce a single summary estimate for a parameter with a confidence interval or summary P value. The method ensures that each study is given appropriate weight according to its power.

The main value of this approach is when many studies of similar design have addressed the same study question, but each individually has low power. In the combined analysis power may be considerably enhanced. Thus a meta-analysis by Yusuf and colleagues, published in 1985, examined the efficacy of long term β blockers in reducing mortality after myocardial infarction. The analysis included data from 24 separate randomised controlled trials, of which only four had shown statistically significant (P<0·05) benefits when analysed individually. In the pooled analysis, however, a clear benefit was apparent, with an estimated 20% reduction in mortality ($P < 0.00001$).

The techniques of meta-analysis work best for randomised controlled trials, which tend to be more uniform in design and suffer from fewer biases than observational studies. An essential requirement is that the criteria for including studies in the analysis be clearly specified at the outset. Otherwise, there is a danger that rules for inclusion will be manipulated consciously or subconsciously to achieve a desired outcome. If the results of a particular study do not conform to the expectation of the investigator, it may be tempting to find a reason to exclude it.

With the inclusion criteria defined, the other crucial element is to ensure that all eligible studies are identified. This may not be easy because not all investigations get published in mainstream journals and some do not get published at all. However, it is a necessary process because the studies that do not achieve prominent publication tend to be those with less interesting (non-positive) results. If they are omitted then the summary assessment will be biased in favour of a positive outcome. A careful search must be made of all available sources of information, including old registers of ongoing research projects and abstracts of reports presented at scientific meetings.

Working with statisticians

Doctors carrying out their own research will often need to seek advice from a medical statistician. It is a good idea to make contact at the planning stage of a study rather than to come later with a mass of data collected in a suboptimal way and ask for help in sorting it out.

When working with a statistician, doctors should try to understand the principles of the analytical method, even if they do not follow all the fine details. In particular, it is important to identify any biological assumptions that are inherent in the analysis and to assess their acceptability.

Summary

The techniques of statistical inference help us to interpret the findings of studies, but the results of statistical calculations do not on their own determine medical decisions. Like the results of laboratory tests, they must be interpreted in context. Sensible interpretation is possible even if the mathematics underlying the calculations is not fully understood. This book has tried to introduce the principles of statistical analysis in a way that clinicians will find practical and relevant. Readers who wish to explore the subject in more detail should consult the recommendations for further reading on page 112.

Answers

Chapter 1

1.1 (a) Continuous quantitative.

(b) Continuous quantitative.

(c) Discrete quantitative.

(d) Nominal (the categories of blood group have no natural order).

(e) Discrete quantitative (there are only eight possible values for the titres).

(f) Nominal.

(g) Ordinal (there is a natural sequence from primary through secondary to higher).

(h) Discrete quantitative (unless the patients were extremely promiscuous, in which case the variable might be treated as continuous quantitative).

(i) Nominal.

(j) Nominal (the categories have no natural order).

(k) Ordinal.

1.2 Six: sex × age, sex × presenting complaint, sex × medication, age × presenting complaint, age × medication, presenting complaint × medication.

Chapter 2

2.1 (a) No. HLA type is a nominal variable; histograms are used for continuous quantitative variables.

(b) No. Few surgical units would carry out more than 20 appendicectomies in a week, so this would normally be treated as a discrete quantitative variable and summarised graphically by a bar chart.

(c) Yes. Concentration of γ-glutamyl transferase is a continuous quantitative variable.

(d) No. This is a discrete quantitative variable.

2.2 (a) Yes. The number of filled teeth in a child must be a whole number between 0 and 20. Thus it is a discrete quantitative variable and a bar chart could be used.

(b) Yes. As defined, the result of smear testing is an ordinal variable with three values. A bar chart could therefore be used.

(c) No. Peak flow is a continuous quantitative variable, so a histogram would be used rather than a bar chart.

(d) No. Serum amylase activity is a continuous quantitative variable.

2.3 (a) Yes. This is a discrete quantitative variable.

(b) Yes. This is a continuous quantitative variable.

(c) No. Grade of retinopathy is an ordinal variable.

(d) Yes. Amount spent is a continuous quantitative variable.

2.4 (a) False. It is symmetrical.

(b) True.

(c) True. This follows from the symmetry of the distribution.

Chapter 3

3.1 (a) Contingency table or bar chart (nominal × nominal data).

(b) A table or graph showing summary measures of central tendency and dispersion for length of stay across different values of Glasgow coma score (ordinal × discrete quantitative). A dot plot might also be possible.

(c) A table or graph showing summary measures of central tendency and dispersion for IQ across different values of APGAR score, or a dot plot (ordinal × continuous quantitative).

(d) Contingency table or bar chart (nominal × ordinal).

(e) Contingency table or bar chart (fatality is nominal (fatal or not) and day of week is ordinal).

(f) Scatter plot and possibly a correlation coefficient or regression line (both variables are continuous quantitative).

(g) Contingency table (for each surgeon, diagnosis is a nominal variable with two categories—direct and indirect).

Chapter 4

4.1 His father does not have the disease, and therefore cannot carry the gene. It follows that his sister must have acquired the gene from their mother and the mother must carry the gene. The mother must be a heterozygote since if she were a homozygote she would pass on a defective gene to all her children and his brother would also have the disease. It follows that the man has a 50% probability of inheriting a defective gene from his mother and of having the disease.

4.2 Let us assume that the surgeon sees 1000 patients, of whom 250 have appendicitis. Of the 250 with appendicitis, he will correctly diagnose $250 \times 88\% = 220$. Of the 750 without appendicitis he will correctly exclude the diagnosis in $750 \times 86\% = 645$. It follows that he will incorrectly diagnose appendicitis in $750-645 = 105$ patients. Thus, altogether he will diagnose appendicitis in $220 + 105 = 325$ patients, of whom 220 will actually have the disorder. The predictive value of his diagnosis of appendicitis is therefore $220/325 = 67 \cdot 7\%$.

True diagnosis	Surgeon's diagnosis		
	Appendicitis	Not appendicitis	Total
Appendicitis	220	30	250
Not appendicitis	105	645	750
Total	325	675	1000

In making this calculation, a sample of 1000 patients was assumed in order to make the arithmetic simple, but (aside from any rounding errors) the same predictive value would be obtained if we assumed a sample of a different size.

4.3 (a) The probability that a true case is positive on electrocardiography is 80% and the probability that a true case is positive on cardiac enzymes is 65% (from the given sensitivities). As the two tests are independent, the probability that a true case is positive on both tests is obtained by multiplying these probabilities: $80\% \times 65\% = 52\%$.

(b) The probability that a true case will be positive for either one or both tests is the sum of the probabilities of being positive on each test separately minus the probability of being positive on both tests: $80\% + 65\% - 52\% = 93\%$.

(c) The probability that a non-case will be negative on electrocardiography is 50% and the probability that a non-case will be negative on cardiac enzymes is 65% (from the given specificities). Since the two tests are independent, the probability that a non-case will be negative on both tests is obtained by multiplying these probabilities: 50% × 65% = 32·5%.

(d) The probability that a non-case will be negative for either or both tests is the sum of the probabilities of being negative on each test separately minus the probabilities of being negative on both tests: 50% + 65% − 32·5% = 82·5%.

(e) In this situation the sensitivity is the probability that a true case is positive on both tests (52%) and the specificity is the probability that a non-case is negative on either or both tests (82·5%).

(f) In this situation the sensitivity is the probability that a true case is positive on one or both tests (93%) and the specificity is the probability that a non-case is negative on both tests (32·5%).

Chapter 5

5.1 (a) Rates of wound infection are the same with the new surgical technique as with conventional treatment.

(b) The average waiting time for an outpatient appointment is the same for patients from fundholding general practices as from other general practices.

(c) In children with middle ear disease rates of absence from school are the same after adenoidectomy as in comparable children who have not had the operation.

5.2 (a) If in general the new analgesic produced no better or worse pain relief than conventional treatment, the probability of observing a difference in pain relief between the new analgesic and conventional treatment as large as or larger than that found in the trial would be 0·02 (2%).

(b) If the underlying workloads of the two departments were identical, the probability of finding a difference between them in numbers of hip fractures treated over 12 months as large as or larger than that observed in the study would be more than 0·05 (5%).

(c) If advice not to leave babies face down in their cots had no influence on rates of sudden infant death, the probability of observing a difference in the rates of sudden death as large as or larger than that found in the study would be less than 0·05 (5%).

Note that in each of the above examples, the definition of the P value starts with an "if."

Chapter 6

6.1 (a) Assuming that there was no bias in the study method, the true ratio of leukaemia mortality in men who participated in nuclear weapons tests is likely to be between 1·01 and 3·06 times that in the comparison group from which the controls were selected. If the true ratio were outside this range, the probability of obtaining results as or more extreme than those observed would be less than 5% (0·05).

(b) Yes. If there were no underlying differences in mortality rates from leukaemia in the study group and controls, the ratio of their rates would be one. One lies outside the range 1·01 to 3·06. Therefore, if the null hypothesis of no underlying difference in rates were correct, there would be less than a 5% probability of finding a difference as large as or larger than that observed.

6.2 (a) Assuming that there was no bias in the trials analysed, the true efficacy of nicotine chewing gum in people of the sort studied is likely to lie somewhere in the range 4% to 8%. If the true efficacy were outside this range then there would be less than a 5% probability of obtaining results as or more extreme than those found.

(b) By studying larger numbers of people.

Chapter 7

7.1 General practice age–sex registers, school registers.

7.2 If there is a limit on the availability of cases then the power of a study can be increased by having more than one control per case, but there is a law of diminishing returns and it is not worth going beyond a ratio of four or five to one unless additional controls can be obtained very easily and cheaply.

7.3 One would start by specifying a benefit from therapy worth detecting, perhaps a 20% improvement according to an appropriate measure. The power of the study would then be expressed as the probability of its finding a statistically significant (normally at a 5% level) difference in outcome between treated patients and controls if treatment conveyed a benefit of this specified magnitude. Thus, if therapy produced a 20% improvement, the study might have an 80% probability of obtaining a statistically significant difference between treated patients and controls.

7.4 A confidence interval around an estimate of the benefit from therapy.

7.5 The relevance of the smoking habits of the two occupational groups lies in the possibility that they might contribute to differences in lung cancer rates between the groups. The potential contribution depends on the magnitude of any difference in smoking habits rather than its statistical significance. The statistical significance depends on the numbers of subjects as well as the magnitude of the difference in their smoking habits. A large difference might not be statistically significant if the number of subjects was small, but it would still be important in this context.

Chapter 8

8.1 The nature of the treatments might be such that any differences in risk of death would be expected to apply only in the short term (for example, before patients have mobilised). In this case, the assumption of a constant ratio of mortality risks at all intervals since the start of treatment would be questioned.

Further reading

Altman DG. *Practical statistics for medical research.* London: Chapman and Hall, 1991.

This book is aimed primarily at medical researchers with limited previous exposure to statistics teaching. It is also useful to medical students and doctors who want more than just an introduction to the subject.

Armitage P, Berry G. *Statistical methods in medical research.* Oxford: Blackwell, 1993.

An excellent source of reference for the more mathematically inclined.

Bland JM. *An introduction to medical statistics.* Oxford: Blackwell, 1987.

Aimed at medical students and doctors, but it helps if the reader is comfortable with algebraic formulas.

Campbell MJ, Machin D. *Medical statistics—a commonsense approach.* Chichester: Wiley, 1993.

The more complicated mathematics is kept in an appendix, making the book relatively easy to read.

Coggon D, Rose G, Barker DJP. *Epidemiology for the uninitiated.* London: BMJ Publishing Group, 1993.

A concise introduction to epidemiology covering study design and interpretation.

Gardner MJ, Altman DG. *Statistics with confidence.* London: BMJ Publishing Group, 1989.

This book concentrates particularly on the rationale for using confidence intervals in statistical inference and the techniques for calculating them.

Pocock SJ. *Clinical trials—a practical approach.* Chichester: Wiley, 1983.

A thorough and readable account of the methods used in clinical trials.

Swinscow TDV. *Statistics at square one.* 8th ed. London: BMJ Publishing Group, 1983.

A short guide for those wanting to carry out simpler statistical analyses for themselves.

Index